Camille's Children

Camille's Children

31 MIRACLES AND COUNTING

Camille Geraldi

and

Carol Burris

Andrews and McMeel

A UNIVERSAL PRESS SYNDICATE COMPANY

KANSAS CITY

Library of Congress Cataloging-in-Publication Data

Burris, Carol and Camille Geraldi.
    Camille's children : 31 miracles and counting / by Camille Geraldi and Carol Burris.
        p.   cm.
    Includes bibliographical references.
    ISBN 0-8362-2144-3 (hd)
    1. Geraldi, Camille.   2. Up with Down Syndrome Foundation.
3. Mentally handicapped children—Florida—Family relationships—
Case studies.   4. Down's syndrome—Florida—Case studies.
5. Special needs adoption—Florida—Case studies.   6. Mothers—
Florida—Biography.   7. Family—Florida—Case studies.   I. Title.
HV897.F6B87   1996
362.4'043'083—dc20   96-4065
                                                                CIP

DEDICATION

Such an unusual dedication page for such an unusual family. My heart tells me to dedicate this book to my husband, Michael, whose everlasting love has always allowed me to follow my dream. But the love and gratitude in my heart increase with each day, so I must include many others.

To Renae and Jaclyn, my precious biological daughters. Without their love for me and our family, this would never be.

To all my beautiful children, each of them so special in so many ways: Darlene, Tiffany, Champ, Woody, Mariah, Karley, Courtney, Seth, Jo-Layne, Brooke, Matthew, Adelle, Kellie-Ann, Kyle, Christopher, Derrick, Joelle, Sandriana, Camia, Michael, Sarah, Adam, Sonny, Angelica, Cookie, Meredith, Jahida, Carmelo, Sophie, Janeece, Jackson, Samantha, Funky, Rahat, Marian, Jaxie, Agnes, Shanti, Luigi, Luis, and Donovan. They are my inspiration.

To my extended family: Penny, Henry, Sheba, Rick, Sarah, Michelle, Tricia, Wendy, Leanne, Joanne, Marci, Eric, and John. Each of them has the same devotion to the children that I have.

To my mother, Ann. Over the years she has learned to look at and love all her grandchildren, to accept and respect this path I have chosen, and to nurture and encourage me as if I were her little girl again. In doing so, she has taught me unconditional love.

And last but not least, to my father, Tony. He never understood my weight or my love for people less fortunate, but even though he withheld his praise and support, he taught me the most precious gift in life—to share, to care, and to love no matter what obstacles stand in the way.

—Camille Geraldi

I owe this book, my sons, my life, and my passion for Baby Ruth's to Butch Burris.

He already owns my heart.

—Carol Burris

Contents

. . . .

. . . .

ACKNOWLEDGMENTS

To all the parents who have trusted me over the past three years to love each one of their children as if tha was the only one I had. Their struggles, along witl confidence and faith in me, is what this book is all al parenting.

With all the love in my heart, I must say that with devoted sister Jo-Ann constantly by my side handl paperwork, legal issues, and everlasting phone ca book would never be.

Rosemary, my perfect rose who never wilts, alv tient, always calm, and always on the computer every thought. Her dream is that someday I will turn the computer on.

Bill, my constant companion, friend, and board. Without his caring for the children and for dation, without his devotion to me, I would ne peace of mind. Nor would I have the beautiful p my family to carry into eternity. It is so cute when first words from one of the children is "Cheese!"

And finally to Carol—for believing in my lifelo for seeing my vision, and for wanting to write a b it. She has inspired me to never stop reaching for I love you, Carol, for giving yourself to all our li always believing in me.

—Camille G

The work on this book, the soul-satisfying,
life-altering labor of this book, was made possible by
three rare and powerful women who held my head
above water until I learned to swim:
Marilynn McCormick, Jane Flanagan and Pat Hamer

—Carol Burris

Introduction by Carol Burris

❧

One Sunday evening, I was watching *60 Minutes* as Lesley Stahl interviewed Camille Geraldi, the mother of nineteen sick, handicapped children. Moved by the matter-of-fact way Camille talked about her family, I wanted to make a contribution to her work. Perhaps I could write a book and donate the royalties to her non-profit organization. I wrote to her the next day.

She responded within a week and invited me to Florida. I was delighted even though I had some questions. Did Camille and her husband have any ulterior motives when they took the children in? What did Camille get out of it? Money? Celebrity? And how could you rear that many children and still love and nurture each one of them as an individual? I had also never been around handicapped children or spent any time with a child who was extremely ill. Scared to death, I flew to Florida.

Camille and I hit it off immediately, but my first in-

troduction to the children was not what I had expected. Many of them were born with Down syndrome, and they share certain facial characteristics. As
a result, when six or seven of them bounced into the
room together, they all looked alike to me. And I
couldn't understand a word they said.

The only one who stood out was a scowling little boy
about four named Champ. I waited nervously as he
marched toward me and planted himself directly in
front of my chair. Then he laughed, leaned his elbow
on my knee, and kissed me on the cheek. At that moment, I was his, and this book was born.

Over the next two years, I spent so much time with
the Geraldi family that it felt as if I were a member of
the family. Combining the talents of General Patton
and Mother Teresa, Camille supervised a husband,
two biological daughters, nine live-in staff members,
four adults with special needs, not to mention all the
children. Yet, they treated one another as true family.

Anyone who is skeptical should visit them, unan-
nounced. So should the doctors and nurses who might
question Camille's authority or her knowledge. Like
many mothers, she has been refused admittance to examination rooms, ignored by nurses who resent her
tending to her own children, and patronized by doctors unwilling to consider her wisdom.

I wrote the book in the first person, because I
wanted you to hear Camille's voice as I do. And while

the book is about her family, it is also about parenting. Camille applies her philosophy of love and discipline to all children. She says there is nothing unusual in what she does. In her eyes, raising these children doesn't make her special. It simply makes her a human being.

You won't forget her or the children. How many are there today? Thirty-one and counting.

1 *A New Baby*

❧

"We're getting another baby!" I yelled excitedly, and slammed down the receiver.

Five minutes earlier, the furthest thing from my mind was a new baby. I had been sitting in the backyard, writing a thank-you letter and watching my toddlers play in their wading pool. Jaclyn, one of my teenagers, was leading them in a group sing.

"One little, two little, three little Indians. Four . . . Come on, Adelle, sing." Jaclyn tickled Adelle's foot and laughed.

That was when the phone rang. I motioned to the children to be quiet and picked up the receiver. "Up With Down Syndrome Foundation, Camille Geraldi speaking." I signed my name to the thank-you letter and reached for an envelope as the voice on the line introduced himself and began to speak. Suddenly my hand froze in midair. This man was asking me if I wanted to adopt another baby.

I answered quickly before he could change his mind. "Of course, of course, we'll take it," I cried, overjoyed at the request.

. . . .

The thank-you letter lay forgotten in front of me as my mind raced ahead to next month's schedule and the plans that had to be made for this new arrival. The minute the call ended, I jumped up and rushed into the house to tell my sister Jo-Ann and the rest of the staff. "We're getting another baby! It's only a week old."

"Wait! Mom!" Jaclyn shouted. "Come back, I want to hear too."

"I'll be right back," I yelled over my shoulder. As I searched for my staff, I asked myself a dozen questions. Did I have enough new-baby clothes? And where had I seen that advertisement for a brass cradle? Most important, how busy was my schedule in the months ahead? I always keep a new baby with me every minute of the first six months to make sure we bond.

Months ago, we lost an infant, and I had been devastated. When it happened, I told my husband, Mike, no more babies, no more for a long time. And we had gotten only one call until now. Then this one, out of the blue. Things happen for a reason, I always say.

I hurried down the hall, through the living room and past the kitchen, to the playroom, the heart of the house. We have three houses on this block, half an hour from Miami—one my husband and I own, another the foundation owns, and a third one that we rent. (Our neighbors have tolerated us well over the years, while we, in turn, are careful to keep the noise level down, especially on weekends.)

All three of the houses' backyards butt up against one an-

other to form one large backyard. To keep people from getting confused, we refer to each house by its color: pink,
purple, or blue. In the pink house, where my office is, the
children are dressed and fed. They sleep in the purple
house, and we keep the blue one for the clerical staff. Living in three different houses sounds strange to some people, but it isn't once you get the hang of it.

We need every bit of the space too. As the head of the Up
With Down Foundation, I organize and direct a crew of nine
live-in staff members, 350 volunteers, and six handicapped
adults who also live and work here with us. These adults with
special needs and the staff are like family to me, a family that
includes my pediatrician husband, Mike; our two biological daughters, Renae and Jaclyn; and thirty adopted handicapped children. Yes, you heard me right, thirty, soon to be
thirty-one.

For years, we have taken in only seriously ill handicapped
children. I also counsel parents with handicapped children,
provide respite care for families that need some time off,
and teach new parents the early intervention techniques that
we use here at the foundation.

"Jo-Ann! Where did everybody get to? Where are you?
You won't believe it. Who did I just hear say it was time for
a baby again?"

I heard the kids' voices. Of course, I should have realized, it was lunchtime. They were in the playroom. Standing in the doorway, my hands on my hips, I caught my breath
and surveyed the scene before me. A mural painted by a vol-

unteer covers the walls with pink and yellow hot-air balloons, Disney-green hills, and cartoon bluebirds perched on the branch of a tree.

In the center of the room stood two rows of high chairs with a hungry toddler in each one. The staff and volunteers hurried back and forth, weaving between the children to pick up a spoon, right a cup, or wipe off a dirty face. The children love to eat, and keeping up with their demands at mealtime isn't easy. Karley, one of my four-year-olds with Down syndrome, raised her arms and giggled when she saw me coming.

"Look at you!" I said as I squeezed her cheeks with one hand and tried to straighten the bow on top of her head with the other. The girls hate these bows and yank them out of their hair every chance they get. But I love them.

Karley said something to me, her speech thick and difficult to understand. It didn't help that her mouth was full.

I leaned down and looked her in the eye. "Swallow, Karley. Good. Now say it again, please."

She repeated it, but I still didn't understand. "Does anyone know what she's saying? Karley doesn't seem to care, but I would like to know what my own daughter is talking about." The staff laughed, and Karley, delighted with their noise, laughed and chewed and laughed and reached for more.

"She's asking you where Adelle is," Bill explained. He was standing on the other side of the room with Jo-Ann.

"Oh, there you are. Didn't you hear me yelling? We pick

up a new baby tomorrow. She has Down syndrome, but I don't have all the details yet. So, Jo-Ann, get the paperwork together. Bill, I have someone coming tomorrow at one, so we have to be out of here by nine sharp to pick up the baby and get back on time."

I wiped banana off my daughter's cheek. "Adelle's out back swimming, Karley, because she already ate. When you're done here, you can have a little swim before your nap. Bill, have you got those instructions straight?"

He ducked his head and nodded. Jo-Ann, unfazed by my big surprise, hurried away to go over the adoption papers.

"Another baby! And a newborn at that! I can't wait. Didn't I say we'd get one when it was time?" I turned on my heel and headed back outside. "Wait until Jaclyn hears."

I still couldn't believe it. That made thirty-one children. Holy Moses, when word got out, somebody was going to complain! Whenever we adopted a new child, someone always wrote a letter, or complained to the newspaper, or told us right to our faces that no one, not even the Geraldis, could possibly love that many children. But I loved each one of them as though I had only one. Why wouldn't I?

If a mother had a son, and then two years later had another son, did anyone say, "Oh, how sad. Now her first son will get only half as much love as he used to get." No, of course not. Having a second child doesn't divide and diminish a mother's love the way a mathematician divides and reduces his numbers. Love isn't a pound of meat that can be weighed or a truckload of bricks that can be counted. Love isn't finite and measurable, bound by logical rules. Love is illogical and irrational. It is bottomless. There is plenty to go around, whether there are two children or thirty-one children.

I heard Jaclyn singing before I saw her. You could hear her halfway down the block. "One little, two little, three little Indians." Jo-Layne, Kellie-Ann, Mariah, and Adelle, four- and five-year-old members of the official wading pool glee club, sat in water to their waists, their eyes glued to Jaclyn, while their brothers Seth and Matthew hung out together on the side of the pool. Both boys have dark hair and dark eyes and were more interested in dumping water out of the pool than in singing. All of them have pot bellies, a typical result of Down syndrome, and what they should have been doing was exercising. Most people with Down syndrome, born with poor muscle tone, lead less active lives and burn fewer calories than the rest of us. Diet, while critical, doesn't always overcome the problem.

"Four little, five little, six little Indians . . ."

As Jaclyn sang a number, she held up that many fingers and waggled them in front of the kids. The children, mesmerized, mimicked her every movement.

"Oowa, oowa, shoot the arrow," she sang as she slid her hand down her arm. Four children slid their hands down their arms. Seth joined in too. This was his favorite part.

"Jumped in the boat and the boat tipped over." Jaclyn slapped the water with the palm of her hand and showered water everywhere. The kids laughed and splashed each other.

Jaclyn blew the hair out of her eyes and paused. "Seth?" She glanced at him and flicked something off his cheek. "A leaf? What did I tell you? Quit eating leaves." She turned back to her glee club. "Tiffany, ready?"

On Jaclyn's left, Tiffany lay on her belly, resting on the bottom of the pool. Our six-year-old tomboy, she had been waiting patiently for her cue. Her orange bathing suit flashed in the sun as she held her chin above water and nodded.

"Go!" Jaclyn yelled.

"Sthwim, sthwim, sthwim, little Indian," Tiffany gurgled as she dog-paddled across the little pool. I winced at her lisp. I hoped once the rest of her front teeth came in, she'd sound more like a little girl and less like Mike Tyson. It felt as if we had been waiting forever for those teeth.

Jo-Layne watched quietly and patted her hands in time to the music.

Jaclyn leaned toward her. "Go, Jo-Layne. Ma-ri-ah."

Jo-Layne watched Jaclyn's mouth and rocked in the pool. Water beaded on her face. Her hair twisted in tangles on her neck. Beside her, Tiffany sang to herself, "Ma-ri-ah."

"La, la, la, la," Jaclyn sang softly, her face a foot from Jo-Layne's. She spotted me coming across the yard and raised her eyebrows, but she didn't stop what she was doing. "La, la . . ."

Moving to the rhythm of the song, Jo-Layne nodded her head slightly, as if saying, yes, I know that one. I remember that song.

"Come on, sing," Jaclyn urged, her eyes wide and expectant. "La, la . . ."

Jo-Layne mouthed the words and patted the air in time to the music.

"That's it. La, la, la, la."

With thick, mumbled words, so soft they were only a whisper, Jo-Layne tried. "Luh."

"La, la, la, la," Jaclyn sang clearly and quietly, so close now that their noses touched.

"Luh, luh, luh, luh," Jo-Layne sang. She sat bolt upright, shocked, surprised at herself.

"Yeah!" Jaclyn cried softly, then grabbed her in a crushing wet hug. "Look, everybody, Jo-Layne's singing."

*F*or many years, Jo-Layne had never sung. Born to a thirty-eight-year-old mother, Jo-Layne arrived in the world with heavy burdens. Her face was bruised and puffy from the difficult breech birth, and she showed all the signs of Down syndrome. She also had a lung disorder, a severe heart defect, and an imperforate anus (no anal opening). Because her mother was unable or reluctant to raise her, the hospital called me. When Jo-Layne was four days old, she required a colostomy, a surgical procedure that creates a canal from the colon to the outside of the body. Five days later, doctors performed another surgery at the site of the colostomy. Then sepsis—staph infection—set in. After that was under control, she had open-heart surgery. Doctors told us she would probably be blind and deaf. They held little hope. They were sure she would be nothing but a vegetable.

Well, she was neither blind nor deaf, and it wasn't long before she was waddling around here, belly out, feet flat, like a pregnant old lady. Her nickname is Jo-Pain, and with all her surgeries and hospital stays, she has earned it. I owe my gray hair to this child.

Now after a year in the hospital following open-heart surgery, she was just beginning to catch up. Quiet and solemn, she was a paler version of her brothers and sisters who sang and danced and bounced around. She wasn't frail as much as slow, slower to move, as if moving required more energy and vigor from her than the others. Jo-Layne is tough though, like I was. Life is a struggle right now, but she'll get through it. She can withstand anything. I did.

I had survived an obese childhood and a critical, temperamental father who hated that I was fat. It was hard growing up with a parent who always yelled at me. But today I am living proof of the saying What Doesn't Kill You Makes You Strong. I am also a different kind of parent to my children than my father was to me. I never yell at the kids, and when I am in a bad mood, I take it out on Mike or my regular staff. They understand my frustrations and put up with me. But I never take it out on the children or the Down syndrome adults. Never.

I learned another important lesson after my painful hysterectomy. Jo-Layne's surgery and her slow recuperation were, like mine, only a moment in time. I had endured my pain, and it had passed and made me stronger—as it would her. I carried that belief in my heart.

2 *Dr. Mike*

✿

*T*hat night after all the excitement about the new baby had died down, my husband, Mike, relaxed next to me on the couch. He's a good man; nice looking, too, with a Roman nose and graying hair he wears clubbed at the nape of his neck. "This is okay with you?" he asked. "This new baby? I thought you didn't want one for a while."

"It's more than okay with me." I smiled to reassure him. My husband is a good man. "It's what I want. But it reminds me of the old days when we couldn't adopt a child for anything."

I met Mike in 1973 at Variety Children's Hospital in Miami when I was a pediatric nurse and he was still an intern. One day he just walked onto the ward where I was working and asked for me. "I came to see this nurse my young patients are always telling me about. Who's Aunt Camille?"

I smiled and introduced myself. I had heard the other nurses talking about the cute, young Italian doctor, but he and I hadn't met. We exchanged a few words, he left, and I didn't expect to see him again. Actually, I really didn't think about it. After all, I was still fat. At that point in my life, I weighed 325 pounds and seldom thought about dating.

One night I stayed at the hospital after my shift was over to sit with a terminally ill infant. Isabelle was born with spina bifida (exposed spinal cord) and other abnormalities so severe she had only a few days to live. I was leaning over her incubator that night, my chin on my arm, watching her as she slept when the door opened and Mike walked in.

He looked surprised to see me. "What are you doing here? Don't you work days?"

"I do. I just wanted to spend some time with Isabelle. She's not doing very well."

He watched us quietly for a while. "You really love her, don't you?"

"Of course, I do. I've always taken care of children like her on my own time," I said with a quick glance up at his face. "My father used to give picnics for handicapped people, and I've worked with them all my life. The ones nobody else wants, they're my life. Besides, Isabelle was my first patient in pediatrics.

"I was so scared. Then when I saw her, all the fear left me, and I fell in love with her immediately. Now she's dying, and I won't let her die alone. That's why I'm here."

"I saw you outside today with some of them," Mike said. "Do you always do that?"

I nodded. "Every chance I get. Do you know some of the children live here as boarder patients, and they've never seen the sky or touched the grass? Do you understand? They've never watched the rain fall or felt the wind in their faces—" I shut up. I didn't want him to think I was some kind of nut.

"I know how you feel about these kids. I feel the same way. I've wanted to be a pediatrician my whole life." As he gazed at Isabelle, he asked softly, "Next time you take these children outside, can I go with you?"

"Of course," I replied, surprised at the question.

Over that next year, we spent a lot of time together with the children, and a real friendship developed between us. As the months passed, our relationship began to change. One evening we were sitting in front of my friend Dottie's house, and I was talking, like I always did, about how I wanted to raise handicapped kids, when Mike interrupted me. "I want to do it with you."

"Sure," I said with a shrug. "I'm really going to need a good pediatrician, and . . ."

"I don't mean it that way," he said, his face serious.

Wait a minute, I thought to myself. What's he saying to me?

"We were meant to be married, Camille."

What? Did he just ask me to marry him? Was that a proposal? I knew everyone at the hospital had been wondering what was going on, and I had asked myself some of the same questions. But me, the fat nurse, with the doctor every other nurse was after? I had never thought about marriage. I never expected to find anyone who would want to raise these children with me.

Mike's eyes searched my face for my reaction. When he saw

me open my mouth, he knew what I was going to say, and he held up his hand. "I don't see your weight, Camille," he said, reading my mind. "I see something else. I see your compassion and your love. I see your commitment and your determination. They're the things I see and love in you." He smiled. "You just need a big body to hold that big heart of yours."

He saw whatever quality I had that drew me to these children and them to me. He saw whatever quality I had that most people, even my father, didn't see. Here was a doctor who could have had it all, and he wanted to be part of *my* life. With all those other women Michael Geraldi might have picked, who would have thought Camille Martone would be the lucky one?

We were married in 1975. But between you and me, I think he got a little more than he bargained for. Being a pediatrician was not the same thing as being a father to thirty-one children. That was never his dream. But after we were married, he willingly became our sole support, and his salary allowed me to live out my dream. He made it all possible. Through the years, he has spent over $800,000 on my children. So don't ever think I am the saint in the family. The saint is Michael.

Still, those early days were hard. Not because of money. I helped in Mike's office, and his pediatric practice grew. In 1977, I gave birth to two daughters, Renae and Jaclyn, born only ten months apart. Life for the Geraldis was easy. I had a lovely home and a swimming pool. Dr. Mike drove a Porsche, and I had a Mercedes. We owned a boat and a

. . . .

motor home, and I had all the jewelry I could want. Money was definitely not a problem.

But the births of the girls and the busyness of our lives sidetracked me. When I saw how bored and unfulfilled I was, I realized it was because I wasn't doing what I had planned to do with my life. I had known my purpose since I was in grade school. There was a girl the kids made fun of because of the way she acted. They called her retarded. I didn't know what that meant until I asked my mother.

"The kids don't like her," I said in tears. "How come nobody wants to play with her?"

"I don't know, but you can't make them like her." She held my chin in her hand and watched my face as she explained. "She's not retarded. She has a tumor in her head. That's why she acts funny. That's why she drags her foot when she walks. She just can't help it."

"That's so sad," I cried.

"Yes, I know it is, but these things happen. They happen to a lot of people."

"Can I catch it?"

My mother smiled slightly and shook her head as she pulled me in for a hug.

I'll make friends with her I decided, and I did. A year later, she died. From that time on, people with handicaps were especially important to me.

By the time Renae and Jaclyn were eight and nine, it was 1986, and I was applying to every adoption agency I could find, adding my name to each waiting list, including Florida's Department of Health and Rehabilitative Services. I explained that I wanted handicapped children, children with neurological deficits so medically involved that they were incompatible with life. I pointed out time and again that Mike was a pediatrician, and I was a nurse. We knew how to take care of these children.

For years we waited, but nothing happened.

Finally, the Down Syndrome Adoption Exchange in White Plains, New York, called. I couldn't believe it, a child in Mississippi was available for adoption. As soon as we heard, we left to bring our new daughter home. Born in March 1986, and only five weeks old, she weighed barely four pounds and was profoundly handicapped. She was a half-Indian, half-black, Down syndrome baby. Very few facts about her background were available. All we really knew was that her mother was a full-blooded Cherokee who had been raped by a black man. After the baby's birth, the mother quickly abandoned her.

The baby was the color of café au lait, and her funny ears jutted out on either side of her little face like handles on a soup bowl. I named her Darlene. She was my first adopted child. I have to chuckle when I think about it now. We were so ignorant of the adoption process that we crossed state lines illegally while bringing her home. Of course, we had no idea at the time that we needed to be represented by an attorney who would file for permission for us to take her out of the state. But, oh, we learned a lot after that.

Darlene was so severely, profoundly retarded that she appeared autistic. She seemed unreachable. She couldn't hear, couldn't drink, and every time we fed her, she spit up most of her formula. The doctors called her a failure-to-thrive baby, but I didn't agree. I had such fun with her. She brought me so much joy. They didn't think she would ever be able to stand. But she did. Before she was two, she stood by herself in her crib. When she was three, she taught herself to swim. Almost.

I was floating around in our backyard pool one afternoon, talking to Renae while she played with Darlene on the grass ten yards away from the edge of the pool's concrete walk. Without warning, Darlene turned and headed in my direction. Renae flew after her as I yelled, "Grab her! Renae, get her!"

Darlene never looked back. She just smiled and dashed toward me. Picking up speed, she raced across the concrete walk, never stopping at the edge of the pool. She just ran right out into the water six feet from where I stood. As her feet left the ground, her legs windmilled wildly in the air, but she made no sound. I screamed and grabbed for her as she hit the water. I missed, and Darlene sank like a stone.

In seconds, I dove to the bottom of the pool and reached for her. The blood thumped in my ears, and my muscles stiffened with fear. Yet when I pulled Darlene through the water toward me, her muscles remained relaxed, pliant. It seemed to take forever to get to the surface with her, but she never tried to hang on to me or break away in a panic. She didn't know enough to be alarmed.

When our bodies broke the surface, she grinned while water streamed out of her mouth. The plunge never fazed her. Darlene didn't know the difference between water and air. Thank heaven, she was all right. She turned six on her last birthday. We nicknamed her Dar Dar and watch her like a hawk around water.

Tiffany, our toothless swimmer, arrived next. Born in 1987 to a couple from New York, Tiffany was diagnosed at birth with Down syndrome. Because there were no medical problems, the family opted for respite care. (Respite care provides a breather for parents who need some time to themselves.) When the respite provider became too busy to continue to care for Tiffany, we were called. Mike and I picked her up in Atlanta, and, as soon as I held her in my arms, I knew we had trouble.

"Mike, look at this. Look at her breathing. See how rapid it is!"

He leaned closer, dismayed at what he found. "Her chest's retracting. Who said there were no medical problems? Look how hard she has to work to take a breath."

Tiffany spent her first week with us in the hospital for heart surgery. She bounced back quickly, though, and was soon a champion eater, a sloppy one because of her big tongue, but still a champion. I call her Starvin' Marvin.

As she grew, Tiffany, sweet and square-faced, became one

of our highest functioning children. When she was two years old, she could walk, wave good-bye, and respond to discipline. At three, she was placed in a regular school. I was so upset when it didn't work out. I wasn't upset with Tiffany, we were always very proud of her, I was furious with her teacher and with the classroom parents who complained about her. She and I had worked hard to get her ready for public school. Then, all of a sudden, they said she was a discipline problem. I knew better. I had seen how she was treated. Her teacher simply didn't like her.

Within a month of school, Tiffany had regressed severely. I was annoyed at myself for being so surprised. People's reaction to her and to all of my kids is always terrible. I should have expected it, but I didn't. How I cried when they sent her home. My heart broke for her.

*I*n 1987, a phone call from the hospital brought our next child.

"Mrs. Geraldi, we know you have two Down syndrome children, but we have a little boy here . . ."

A boy! I never wanted a boy. What if there were problems with the girls when he got older? Sexual problems. What would I do then?

"Mrs. Geraldi, are you there?"

But how could I leave him in that hospital? On the other hand . . .

"Do you want another one, Mrs. Geraldi? Do you want this little boy?"

Of course, I said yes, and Martin Anthony, Champ to us, came on board. He was the son of a well-known wealthy Peruvian businessman and a beautiful South American model. When his parents discovered at his birth that he had Down syndrome, they wanted no part of him. That taught me that someone could be famous and rich and still walk away from a baby. He wasn't a cute baby, but what a personality. From the get-go, Champ was the Geraldi Latin dynamo. He is such a pistol you can't help laughing. I was certain he was another high-functioning child, but he was so noisy it was hard to tell. A real showboat, he knows when all eyes are on him, and he stomps around flat-footed, chin down, elbows akimbo.

He is always walking up to one of the other kids, grabbing their cheeks affectionately, and kissing them so hard their eyes water. Champ doesn't walk. He swaggers like a Texan in cowboy boots, mugging with his head cocked, showing off for all the world—except when he is with a baby. Then the little tough guy is all tenderness. He's my goodwill ambassador, my representative to the world. Everyone— the press, my family, all our friends—love him. Yet in all these years, he has never had a visitor.

By 1988, we had adopted nine children. At the time, I thought nine was a lot, but then the list really started to grow. Woody, Karley, Courtney, and Seth; Matthew and Kellie-Ann; Joelle, Mariah, Brooke, and Adelle; Kyle and Christopher; Camia, Derrick, and Sandy; Adam and Sonny; Carmelo, Angelica, Jahida and Meredith, and Sophie.

. . . .

Every one of their stories is sad, but some are sadder than others.

Matthew was born in New York in 1989. Dark hair, dark eyes, fair skin, and a couple of freckles. A real Italian leprechaun. His family checked us out thoroughly before Matthew's mother and grandmother flew with him to Orlando. I was to meet them at the airport and pick up the baby right there in the terminal.

As soon as the two women arrived, the grandmother took me aside. "She can't handle it," she explained as she watched her daughter with growing concern. Then she handed Matthew to me, took her daughter by the arm, and quickly steered her away. I watched as they walked across the waiting room. The mother pulled back as if she wanted to stay. I can still see the scene in my mind's eye. As they moved away, the mother started to scream and scream until the sound of her screams rang through the airport. I will never forget it.

Matthew came to us with many problems. His thyroid functioned poorly, and he had a heart defect that might someday require surgery. Born like Jo-Layne without an anus, Matthew's problem was even more extensive than hers. His ostomies—the two permanent openings to the outside of his body—were not at the normal site but on either side of his body. He was so tiny and the colostomy bags so big that I worried constantly about leakage. Night after night, every other hour, I cleaned out those bags. The last thing I wanted was one of them leaking onto his body. The fluids break down skin in no time.

"What are you smiling at?" I asked him one night while I was working on him. He was barely two months old and lying there as if he didn't have a care in the world. "You little devil, is that how you treat your mommy? You don't even answer her when she asks you a question? Now, I ask you, what kind of kid is that?" I grinned down at him and made a face.

Just as I finished, one of the volunteers walked into the room and pinched her nose. "Phew, how can you stand that smell, Camille? Doesn't it bother you?"

"No, in fact, it doesn't," I answered coolly, springing to Matthew's defense. "Where's your compassion? This is no different than when one of the other kids has diarrhea. They don't want to have diarrhea. Do you think Matthew wants this problem? Of course not. He doesn't want to smell like this. But why should he have to suffer because the odor bothers someone else?"

As Matthew grew, even though we took meticulous care of him, the smell worsened. One day he was sent home from school because of the odor. I got the message and I resented it. Were they telling me that if Matthew doesn't smell good, and no matter how clean he is, he isn't socially acceptable? It worried me to death. What were we going to do when he was fifteen? I didn't think the odor would ever go away. How was he going to handle being reprimanded and shunned for something that wasn't his fault?

. . . .

To complicate everything, his heart defect got worse. Although he had already been operated on a dozen times, Matthew now faced open-heart surgery. Why Matthew? I asked myself repeatedly, after all he had been through. It took me a long time to understand that Matthew and I only had that day. Tomorrow would have to take care of itself. I decided not to brood about his future. Let me tell you, it was the right decision. Today, although he still doesn't smell like a gardenia, watching Matthew is more fun than watching TV. Comical and full of life, he is our chair dancer, boogying and bumping in his seat to every song he hears. I'm so glad he's in our lives.

I won't forget Courtney's mother either. She was gorgeous. Just an unmarried eighteen-year-old kid with a new baby, a baby she and the father were going to keep until they learned the infant had Down syndrome. When she asked a nurse at the hospital what to do, the nurse handed her my number. Courtney's mother gathered her courage and made the difficult call.

I visited her in the hospital that day. The baby was a china doll. I loved her on sight. She had a minor heart defect, but the real problem was her eating. Fed through a tube since her birth, Courtney had no idea how to suck or swallow. Because of the feeding tube, she had never needed to know, but she could be taught. I met them again the day they were discharged. Courtney's mother handed the baby to me in the parking lot of the hospital, then ran away sobbing. She was devastated.

The word *devastation* is the only word I ever found that truly describes a parent's emotions. It is the word I use most often when I talk about a family's pain, the pain of giving birth to a Down syndrome child, or the devastation of giving one up. The dictionary describes *devastation* as destruction, havoc, and loss. All the definitions apply.

As Courtney gets older, she reminds me of a little professor. A round-faced blonde, quiet and serious like Jo-Layne, Courtney watches the world with solemn eyes. Mike teases her when she waves good-bye. Courtney always turns her hand toward her face and wiggles her fingers, as if she's waving good-bye to herself. She almost did once.

It was two years ago on Valentine's Day. Courtney, who had always been one of my healthier kids, wasn't feeling well. At one A.M., I gave her a suppository for her fever. We sat together in the big blue recliner, a chair I always sit in when one of the children is sick, and I held her while we dozed on and off. At four A.M., I put her back in her crib in the next room. I have always been a night owl, working while the kids are in bed, so it was unusual for me to catnap more than two or three hours. That night, though, I watched Courtney for a while to make sure she was sleeping peacefully, then when satisfied she was okay, I went to bed and fell into a sound sleep.

Courtney's crib stood at the end of a short row of cribs that runs the length of a wood-paneled wall in one of the bedrooms. Farthest from the door, she was always the last child in line for the morning wake-up call. That morning, when Angela, a staff member, came on duty at six A.M., for some inexplicable reason, she picked Courtney up first. Dusky and lethargic, the child slumped dully against Angela's chest. Alarmed, Angela tightened her grip on Courtney and ran down the hall to our bedroom.

Already awake, Mike took one look at Courtney and leaped out of bed. "Camille! Quick! Courtney looks bad," he cried. He grabbed her out of Angela's arms and rushed down the hall toward the kitchen, Angela right behind him.

I leaped out of bed and ran after them. I heard Mike pelting her with questions.

"You found her like this? In her crib? Did you get any response at all?"

Angela shook her head and replied in short-spoken breaths as she ran.

Mike raced into the kitchen, laid Courtney on the kitchen counter and tilted her head back. "Camille!! Get in here!" he yelled. "Someone call 911."

Henry grabbed the phone and punched in the number. I heard Mike yell again as I rushed into the kitchen.

"Call 911. Call the hospital!"

"I got it, Mike," Henry cried. He spoke a few words to the 911 operator, stabbed at the hang-up button, and punched the hospital's number.

At that moment, Courtney quit breathing. She was blue gray and unresponsive. By that time, I was at her side. Without taking my eyes off her face, I groped for the stethoscope, placed it on her chest, and listened. "No breath sounds," I said. "But there's still a heartbeat. Let's . . ."

Without warning, Courtney's heart stopped. I willed her to breathe, waiting for the stethoscope to telegraph the sound. Nothing! Only silence. I couldn't believe it. She was in full cardiac arrest.

Mike saw my face, and that was all he needed. He placed his mouth over her mouth and nose and started to breathe for her. I laid the heel of one hand at the base of the sternum in the center of her chest, put my other hand over it, and began the rhythmic pushes of CPR. I blotted every thought out of my head and concentrated on what I was doing. Push. One, two, three, four. Her color was awful. Push. One, two, three, four. She was blue and still.

We worked for three minutes. Angela stood off to the side, out of the way, tears running down her cheeks. Henry waited next to her, his face ashen. Courtney's color grew darker with each second. After almost four minutes, there were still no signs of spontaneous breathing. Mike, breathless and distraught, panted and gulped for air. "It's no use, Camille. She's gone."

"No, no, don't stop! She's not gone," I shouted at him. "Keep going."

He bent his head and blew another breath of air into her body, then raised his head to me again. "She's dead, Cooch. This is useless. She's . . ."

"She's not dead," I cried. "Don't say that. There's no reason for her to be dead!"

We worked for another thirty seconds, then thirty more. I heard the ambulance pull up out front as I glanced at Courtney's hands. "Her nail beds, look, they're turning pink."

Sure enough, when the paramedics raced into the kitchen seconds later, Courtney was breathing. We had revived her. I wrapped her in a blanket and carried her past the medics. They ran after me. When I climbed into the back of the ambulance and sat down clutching Courtney, they tried to take her out of my arms.

"No, I'll hold her," I said, drawing her close. "We just resuscitated her. I'm not putting her down."

Young and frustrated, the medic held his hands out in exasperation. "Then what do you need us for, lady?"

"I don't." I started to stand. "I can go in my own car."

He laid his hand on my arm. "It's the rules. She's our responsibility. Come on," he said gently. "I'll take good care of her."

And he did, but the ordeal wasn't over yet. At the hospital, Courtney's heart stopped beating again. Another full cardiac arrest. The doctors resuscitated her, moved her to intensive care, and put her on a ventilator where she remained for three and a half weeks. There was never a diagnosis. Not one of the doctors ever discovered what had happened, and it never happened again.

I have been a nurse for years, and I have never failed to handle any emergency that came along, but that morning when Courtney's heart stopped, mine did too.

3 *Adelle and Kellie-Ann*

🌿

*I*n powder-blue headpieces that looked like ruffled pancakes, my four-year-old daughter Adelle and the other girls in her dance class stood poised, center stage, waiting for the music to begin. As I watched them in their sky-blue tutus and pale tights, soft, satin dancing slippers on their feet, I marveled at how quiet and straight they stood, their little buns of hair bobby-pinned to the backs of their heads.

This was my daughter's first performance, and she didn't know how to be nervous. I was nervous for her. It didn't bother her either that the older girl on her right was so tall that Adelle came only to her hip. Her legs were longer than my daughter's whole body. But Adelle just stood there grinning, cool as a cucumber.

The music started, and the dancers ran forward, four abreast, to the front of the stage, prancing like real ballerinas, almost on their tiptoes. Caught off guard by the music and the other dancers' sudden movements, Adelle paused and glanced around. She hesitated, then walked flat-footed toward the rest of the dancers, two beats behind.

27

Oh God, I couldn't look. Maybe this was asking too much of her. After all, this recital was being held in the auditorium of Miami High School, a huge room with a wide, intimidating stage, and my daughter was not only younger and smaller, she also has Down syndrome. My heart sank as I watched Adelle and listened to the audience around me.

"Oh, she's adorable."

"Look how hard she tries!"

The class lifted their arms in graceful arcs and swept them backward, first one, then the other, in long, slow circles. Adelle raised her arms and windmilled them around and around, so fast the breeze ruffled her headpiece.

"Isn't she the sweetest thing?" The audience tittered and cooed. A few of them must have realized Adelle was handicapped. I heard someone say, "What a shame!"

Her first pirouette, arms extended over her head, just the tips of her fingers touching, rhymed exactly right with the others. And her plié, back straight, knees bent outward, a little awkward at first, turned out fine. Adelle's attention wandered for a second to something she spotted offstage. I held my breath, but she quickly remembered where she was and what she was supposed to be doing. She checked the other dancers to find her place, then fell right in step. The ballerinas held their hands to their hearts. Adelle held her hand to her heart. When they swayed back and forth, Adelle swayed with them. In time, in tune, she was no reluctant shadow now. When they raised their eyes to the ceiling, she did too, picking up speed for the rest of the routine.

Arms up, arms down. Now a pirouette. Look to the right, the left. Dip and twirl. Plié. Again. Another twirl. And again. Adelle never missed a step. She knew the routine cold, knew it so well that she didn't have to watch the others to know what to do. Adelle knew!

At the end, as each dancer dipped in a sweet curtsy, the audience clapped for this one's grace and that one's beauty, and the winning charm of their youth. Call me biased, but I was sure the loudest applause, the very heart of the applause, was for Adelle Geraldi. The other girls were perfect and pretty, but my Adelle was the star. Not because her attention wandered or her tights were wrinkled just above the knee, not because she was cute or because she was handicapped. They cheered the work she had done. They cheered the endless hours she needed to learn the steps, the time she spent with Jaclyn mastering the gestures, listening to the music and memorizing the cues, the effort she had put into practicing and practicing, then rehearsing on stage. They were cheering Adelle above the rest for only one reason. She had earned it.

Adelle was the second of two children born to a healthy mother in her late twenties. Because the first child was normal, and because of the mother's young age, no prenatal testing had been ordered. Adelle was born with Down syndrome, an extremely severe heart defect, and other medical problems so complicated and so numerous the parents couldn't begin to understand.

The first time the parents and I talked they expressed

their fears tentatively, as if hearing them out loud was too painful. They were scared. Raising a sick *and* handicapped baby was something they didn't think they could handle. They worried that keeping her would split the family up, and not keeping her would make them feel guilty. When we said good-bye, it looked, for the moment at least, like they were in a no-win situation. The second time we met, we spent seven hours together while they agonized over what to do. They didn't want to put the baby up for adoption with an agency or a service. The mother was too afraid she wouldn't see Adelle again.

Finally, they decided to leave her with us on a temporary basis in a guardianship under respite care. The mother continued to worry about closed placement, afraid she wouldn't be able to see her once she was with me. I tried to reassure her, explaining that a guardianship is temporary. She listened, her eyes on the floor, and thought quietly about it. Then she asked me to explain again.

She was making the hard decisions. The mother often did. After all, the primary care of the baby is hers. I was glad to see that her husband supported her in everything. That didn't always happen. Eventually, it was decided. They would temporarily leave the infant with us. If they changed their minds later, they could take the baby home. It was a decision I had seen parents arrive at before. It was too awful to consider giving a child up permanently, no matter where the placement. Parents reach their decision in stages in much the same way you test the water in a hot tub.

The night I went to pick up the baby, I knew in my heart that the placement would be permanent. When I saw the look on the mother's face, I knew she thought so too. She already felt the void. Two days later, the father called to check on the baby. The mother didn't come to the phone, but I couldn't have known her heartache. I had never given birth to one of these children.

A few years later, when I glanced back over Adelle's medical chart, I was reminded of how lucky we were to have her. The following incident was one of many. She was only three months old.

Thursday	10/12	Seizures last night.
Friday	10/13	Admitted to Pediatric Intensive Care. Difficulty breathing. Air hungry. Sedated with chloral hydrate to prevent further seizures. Adverse reaction. Switched to morphine. On call for emergency heart surgery.
Saturday	10/14	Remains in ICU. Very sedated. Responds to her name. Baptized today.
Sunday	10/15	On oxygen. Unable to suck.
Monday	10/16	Surgery at 7:00 A.M.
Tuesday	10/17	Remains in heart room. Right arm cyanotic [blue].

Doctors corrected the heart problem, but there were many more. Now, eight surgeries later, Adelle's scar runs like a silver zipper down the center of her chest. But she is still here. *The real winner.* Her biological family visits her, and she is healthy and happy with two sets of parents.

*P*atty, a staff member, and I talked one afternoon while I sat Adelle on the kitchen counter and brushed her teeth. "Brush-a, brush-a, brush-a," I sang, encouraging her to do it herself. She smiled with toothpaste running down her chin. "See, you brush every tooth like this." She put her hand over mine, and we brushed together.

Patty then chased Kellie-Ann into the dining room and hollered back over her shoulder. "She's refused to give me a kiss for weeks. The other day, I was eating a piece of cake. Well, she turns to me and offers me a kiss. Not *too* smart, eh?" Patty tapped her temple with one finger and beamed proudly. She grabbed Kellie-Ann and plopped her down on the couch. In an instant Adelle crawled up beside her sister, and the two girls played their favorite game.

"Eye?" Adelle asked, touching Kellie-Ann's eyelid.

"Eye," Kellie-Ann answered with a blink.

"Nose?" Adelle asked, reaching over and touching her nose. Kellie-Ann shook her head. She had a cold and was already tired of the game. She didn't want to play anymore.

"Nose?" Adelle asked again with a poke to Kellie-Ann's nose. Kellie-Ann didn't answer. "Nose?" Adelle demanded loudly. Kellie-Ann looked at Patty and started to cry. Adelle had poked too hard.

I picked Kellie-Ann up, sat down in a chair, and laid her across my lap. "That's no way for your sister to treat you, is it?" I clapped her on the back like I always do when she has a cold. She loved it. I crooned nonsense words as I worked. "Kellie-Bells, my Kellie-Bells." Her eyes stared as if she were in a trance, and her mouth fell open, slack and relaxed. I thought she was getting better, but I didn't let her appearance trick me. You didn't fool around when these children were sick. They could turn sour on you in a heartbeat.

We learned that lesson again the previous spring when Kellie-Ann had the same croupy cold. We gave her aerosol treatments and oxygen and clapped her every half hour to keep her chest clear. Even though she had been getting better, she still wasn't breathing well. Mike and I were at a meeting in the city one day when things went very wrong.

Eunice was working in the other house while Penny remained with Kellie-Ann. She had been playing quietly in a playpen when suddenly she collapsed. Penny took one look at her face, buzzed Eunice on the intercom, and yelled, "Get over here! It's Kellie-Ann! I have to take her to emergency."

Eunice flew down the walkway to the other house. Penny didn't have time to tell her anything, but she knew as soon as she saw Kellie-Ann that it was bad. Thank God, Rosie was right there in the same room with them.

"I'm not going to make it to Miami Children's Hospital. It's too far," Penny cried. "I'm taking her to Baptist." (It is only minutes away.) There was diarrhea everywhere, so as

Penny and Rosie rushed the toddler out to the car, Eunice grabbed a towel and ran after them. In the daylight, Kellie-Ann's face was gray.

Eunice looked Penny in the eye. "Get there safe, but hurry, Penny. Hurry!"

Penny learned at the hospital that the damage to Kellie-Ann's lungs from her defective heart and the time she had spent on a ventilator when she was very young had left her dangerously susceptible to croup. After drug therapy and a week in the hospital, she was well enough to come home. Eventually, she was fine.

Kellie-Ann's birth followed two normal births. In the delivery room, the doctor, his face grave, carefully checked Kellie-Ann before he turned to the mother and father. "She has all the symptoms," he said.

The baby's father, Larry, spotted tears in the eyes of the delivery room nurse. Every alarm in his body went off. "Symptoms?" he asked. "Symptoms of what?"

"Down syndrome," the doctor replied.

The first time I met Larry, my heart ached. He was a tall brown-eyed man with a five-o'clock shadow. But you should have seen his daughter. She was a little doll with fine blond hair, barely there eyebrows, and two holes in her heart so big they threatened her life. Kellie-Ann was only weeks old when she was transferred to Miami Children's Hospital. By then, Larry understood that the dilemma was his alone. His wife did not want to keep the baby, and his parents, who had raised and known only physically perfect kids, were so devastated that his father hadn't even been to the hospital. Neither had his in-laws.

When he followed someone's suggestion and called me, I heard the despair in his voice right away. "Where are you?" I asked him. "I want to meet with you." An hour later, I walked up to him in the hospital, held my arms out, and hugged him. "What can I do for you?"

"Down syndrome?" he asked me with a stunned, blank look on his face. "Down syndrome? The room at home is all ready for the new baby."

With that, this grown man I hadn't even been introduced to stood in my embrace and cried. This man, fighting like a warrior for his daughter, finally had someone on his side. We sat down right there in the waiting room and talked. He had a lot to tell me, and we talked for a long time.

His wife was afraid of the baby's medical problems. I couldn't blame her. It was a valid fear. Kellie-Ann was very ill.

"But it's not just the medical problems," Larry said. "It's because Kellie-Ann isn't a perfect child. My wife wants to give her up for adoption. Do you know what that means?"

I didn't answer. We both knew what it meant. He would never see her again.

Months later, he told me how he had felt during that first meeting. "I was overwhelmed that you just walked right up to me and bearhugged me. The whole time you were talking to me I'm wondering, what's this going to cost? I'm thinking, this is going to run me about two thousand dollars a month. Then, after you told me you didn't charge any-

. . . .

thing, I started wondering what your motives were. I kept asking myself, what's up with her? What's behind all this?"

By the end of the afternoon, he had decided to leave the baby with us in respite care while he thought about it. Before anything else could be done, though, Kellie-Ann needed surgery, and before she could have the heart surgery, she needed to gain some weight. She weighed six pounds at birth, but because of her medical problems and the feeding tube, she had lost three pounds—50 percent of her body weight. I went there every day and fed her, and I have to admit, I was proud of the results. In six weeks, she gained one and a half pounds.

After her first surgery, we brought her to the foundation. Larry often stopped in to visit her. He sat in the office with me and held her as we talked, watching her sleep. Who could blame him? She had the lightest china-blue eyes with peaches-and-gold skin. When she got tired, she laid her cheek in the palm of her hand and sucked her little finger until she fell asleep.

"My nine-year-old Christina sucked her little finger just like that," he marveled one day. "They look so much alike. Christina and her brother like to come here with me. They're not afraid of these kids. Sometimes I feel guilty not having Kellie-Ann with me, and I feel even guiltier if I don't visit. But when I do get here, God, it's always a relief. And I don't mean just seeing Kellie-Ann. It helps me to talk to you.

"With getting laid off my job, and the divorce and my finances, I was really depressed. I didn't know who to talk to—until I thought of you. After I talked to you, I saw that the job wasn't important, the finances weren't important, and someone born not perfect wasn't important. What is important is how you are with yourself, and how you feel on the inside."

"And family," I said. "The people you love."

"Yeah, you got it," he echoed warmly. "What's important is family and the people you love."

4 Disney World

Early one spring day, shortly before Easter, all of us took off on a mini vacation. We were barely out of Miami, headed north in the foundation's little pink-and-white bus, and already, we were out of control. With more than two dozen children and almost as many adults along, this was going to be a loud, rowdy holiday. Jaclyn, the volunteers, even the staff, were silly with excitement. The children, caught up in the mood, their faces flushed, their hair damp, clapped and laughed at everything.

Champ and Matthew sat side by side in car seats. Everything Champ did, Matthew did, mouthing and mugging for the video camera like vaudeville comics. All they needed were rubber feet and clown noses. Someone turned the radio up, and the sound of an old Bee Gees song filled the bus. It was *Saturday Night Fever* all over again as Champ and Matthew danced in their seats, wiggling their hips, and stabbing the air with two fingers. Midget John Travoltas out to howl on a Saturday night. Only we weren't going to a disco club. We were on our way to Disney World.

Kellie-Ann shared a seat with one of the two-year-olds. With her arm around his shoulders, a pillow across their laps, Kellie-Ann hauled that poor kid up and down, smushing his face in the pillow so many times he had to be dizzy. When she got tired of the game, the two children rested their heads together on the pillow, a breath apart. I was sure he had whiplash.

Later, when I stuck her in the seat with me to give him a break, she and Karley found a volunteer's Walkman and took turns wearing it. As the music filled Kellie-Ann's head, she sat still as a stone, mouth open, spellbound. Karley, unimpressed, reached for one of my ankle bracelets. The kids always play with them. (I wear them not because I love anklets, but because they were Jaclyn and Renae's baby necklaces that I refuse to cut down to fit my wrist.)

In front of us, a young boy about fourteen, so well behaved he had to be one of our new volunteers, perched on the edge of his seat with a Walkman plugged into his ears and a fixed smile on his face. In the seat beside him, Brooke stuck her finger in her nose and stared up at him, checking out his headphones while he pretended she wasn't there.

"Give Mommy a kiss, Karley-Sue." My four-year-old ignored me. "Give me a kiss," I growled as I leaned over and waited, my face smack up against hers. Without a glance in my direction, she kissed me on the eye and waved me away. She was too excited at all the goings-on to bother with Mommy today. I understood. Hadn't I planted myself in the center of the rear seat on purpose? I didn't want to miss anything either. I was having fun watching their fun.

I laughed at Penny as she clowned around up front, and thought how lucky I was. To have all these children was more than I had ever dreamed. And to have help from people like my two girls, Penny, and the others—people who really love these kids—was more than I could have asked. This scene in front of me was everything to me. All the rest—the publicity, the donations, the attention—they are fine. But I am happiest with these people, doing just what we were doing. I must admit, we had to be the loudest vehicle on the highway.

"How can you stand that racket?" Jo-Ann asked me before we left. "I would go crazy."

"It doesn't bother me," I replied. "I don't notice it most of the time." I'm part of these people. I'm not just responsible *for* them. I belong to them, loved by them, and answerable only to them.

"To the ends of the earth . . ." everyone sang. The older girls had sung this song so often we knew it by heart. They waved their hands in the air, swaying them slowly back and forth. In a tie-dyed T-shirt, Karley bounced in her seat, clapping her hands in time to the music. Jo-Layne's head bobbed loosely on her neck as she fought sleep. The rhythm of the wheels was winning, though. She closed her eyes and clapped once, twice, to the music. Her head sunk lower. One more clap and she rested her face on her arm. Another clap, and she was asleep. All around her, music rocked our bus as we rolled on down the road. I laughed out loud at the joy of it.

By early afternoon, things had settled down. The children were sweet and content, the staff relaxed and mellow. "Oh,

happy day . . ." they sang to a tape someone had popped
into the bus's cassette player. It was an old Protestant hymn
we often sang. The kids loved this song and joined in eagerly on their favorite line. "La, la, la, la, la."

Jo-Layne, awake now and raring to go, drew her elbows
back and slapped her hands together, jive-clapping, in time
and in sync as any musician. Her mouth was open and her
face slack, but as she clapped, there was no awkwardness,
no fumbling in her movements. I thought for a second that
they were someone else's arms. "La, la, la, la, la."

Kellie-Ann had surrendered her headphones, and the noise
stunned her into silence. She sat by a window, the sun on
her face, and stared at the passing scenery. Blue eyes, round
and shiny, not Down syndrome eyes, not in this light anyway. A beautiful child with pale hair and pale, porcelain skin.
She has skin so thin and fine that when the sun shone behind her, it turned her skin translucent.

"La, la, la, la, la."

Champ, worn out from all his chair dancing, tucked his
thumb in his mouth and fell asleep. With his seatmate flak-
ing out on him, Matthew redoubled his energy. He bounced
feverishly in his seat, keeping time with his chin, and his little popped eyes rolled around in his head at the effort. Not
at all concerned with Matthew and looking for something
far more interesting to do, Karley stuck her finger down her
throat and gagged herself.

The next morning, sporting fanny packs and diaper bags,
the staff and I shepherded the kids through the entrance to

Disney World. For almost half of them, this was their first trip to Disney World. Tense with excitement, they held tight to the grown-ups' hands and nearly danced out of their shoes.

They wore bright orange Up With Down Syndrome shirts so they would be easily spotted if, God forbid, one of them got lost. I had on a loud, multicolored hat for the same reason. I worried all the time about losing someone. So far, no problems, at least not with the kids. They were on their best behavior. But, it had been a long drive, and at the moment, the grown-ups on my staff were a different story.

"Let's get the rest of the strollers," I said.

Tired from the trip, no one moved. Finally, after yanking out and tucking in, pulling down and buttoning up, adjusting and blowing and wiping, finally, finally, we were ready. But by that time, Adelle was crying and Courtney was asleep. Silent through it all, our stoic Jo-Layne stuck eight of her ten fingers in her mouth, content to endure the day quietly.

"Champ, where are we?" Rosie cried.

"Mickey Mouse!" he yelled excitedly. He tugged Bill's hand to get him going and pulled him toward the Magic Kingdom ahead. Karley, not in her stroller yet, grabbed Champ, pulled him down on the ground, and planted a long kiss on his face. They played Eskimo, nose to nose, and giggled muffled giggles at their silliness.

We walked and wheeled strollers, climbed on and off the rides, until it was time for lunch. Whenever we spotted one of the Disney characters that strolled through the Magic Kingdom, everything in our group came to a halt. The children loved these characters and would not move until they saw them up close.

"Look, there's Eeyore," I cried. Karley pillowed her head against the big gray donkey's stomach, happy to stay there all day. But it was lunchtime and, like an ogre, I pulled her away.

At lunch, Mickey Mouse visited with us. He walked around the table, stopping at each child to touch and hug, teasing and posing for the camera. Karley shook his hand, unafraid, and leaned in for a hug. Brooke didn't know what to do. She couldn't believe it was Mickey Mouse in the flesh. She shrieked with laughter, scrunched her shoulders, and shivered when he laid his hand on her head. But Kellie-Ann was scared to death. The closer Mickey got to her chair, the quieter she got. When he put his hands on her shoulders, she screwed up her face, opened her mouth, and screamed bloody murder. Mickey beat a quick retreat.

Matthew had been watching his sister's reaction, and as Mickey approached him, he waited warily. When Mickey put his hands on Matt's shoulders, the boy's face turned to stone. Don't touch me, Mickey, it said. Later Minnie Mouse breezed into the room, and Matthew grinned when she held his face in her fat white-gloved hands.

We spent the rest of the day pushing strollers filled with tired children and keeping track of the few who walked. If I counted heads once, I counted heads fifty times. By late afternoon, the kids were overstimulated with all the sights and sounds, and the grown-ups were tired of pushing them around. Under a sky that looked more like rain every minute, our little group grew quiet and irritable. Like measles, the bad mood quickly spread.

Suddenly, it started to pour. The strollers had little awnings that protected the children, but the rest of us hadn't brought umbrellas or raincoats. In seconds, we were soaked through to the skin. Even my underwear was wet. We ran toward the entrance, pushing the strollers ahead of us. It was all the way on the other side of the Magic Kingdom.

Ten minutes later, it was still pouring. "Let's go in here," one of the volunteers urged as she stopped and opened the door to a shop.

"No, it's air-conditioned. I'm afraid they'll get sick," I said. "It's warmer out here." I bent down to wipe Brooke's face.

Bill blinked at the rain and pointed toward the parking lot. "Rick and I will get the bus. We'll be back in five minutes."

I nodded and waved him toward the parking lot. "What do you think, Brooke? Five minutes sound right to you?" She just looked at me. "Yep, I agree. We'll be here forever."

Penny and a volunteer stood off to the side, arms folded across their chests. I caught Penny's eye, wrung my ponytail out, and rolled my eyes. "Hey, Penny. Brooke and I just decided those guys won't be back until dark."

The people hurrying by glanced disdainfully at us. I guess we must have looked strange. Some of the kids were so oblivious to the rain and what was going on around them, and with their runny noses and open mouths, they stood out like sore thumbs. Courtney sat in her stroller with wet bangs and drops of water rolling down her cheeks. Her freckled face never showed any expression as the sky rained down on her.

I wondered where all of the people with Down syndrome were. In that whole day at Disney World, I could have counted the number I saw on one hand. Where were they? Genetic defects are very common, yet where were they all? One in eight hundred births results in a Down syndrome child. Where were those millions of children? I knew where. Parents didn't take them out. When Down children get older, many of them become more stubborn and difficult. Some parents are afraid they'll be embarrassed in public. So they stop taking them anywhere. Why do you think I want to make a home for them?

How people treat us angers me, although I don't show it. Salespeople are rude, teenagers holler uncouth remarks, and strangers ask impolite questions. One day in a mall, a woman approached me as I was window-shopping with one of the babies in my arms. The woman walked right up to me and lifted a corner of the baby's blanket.

I stood there as the woman peered at the baby. I thought perhaps she was one of the people who had seen me before and felt she knew me. (Sometimes people I don't know act as if they are part of my family.) I opened my mouth to ask her name when she dropped the corner of the blanket back over the baby and stared up into my face. Caught off guard, I smiled.

The woman didn't say a word. She just turned and walked

away, nodding to herself. I stood there rooted to the spot, shocked at her nerve.

"I thought you were the one," she called back over her shoulder.

When I calmed down and collected myself, I realized what she had been doing. That woman had recognized me and was checking to see if the baby had Down syndrome. That's why I always insist that my children are neat, clean, and on their best behavior. I want to make them socially acceptable so the rest of the world feels at ease around them. I want them presentable, so the rest of the world stops ridiculing and fearing them. You cannot learn about something you refuse to go near.

I wiped Courtney's face while the children who had been lifted out of their strollers splashed flat-footed in the puddles. Delighted with this new entertainment, they babbled and crowed. In the din, you had to wonder what they were talking about. And here I was, in charge of this outfit, with my hair hanging in my face and my T-shirt wet enough to see through. I tried to think. We couldn't go in air-conditioning. It was too cold. We couldn't wait under a tree. I had heard thunder. We just had to tough it out until Bill came back with the bus. Champ sucked at the neck of his wet T-shirt. Beside him, Brooke stuck her head out from under her stroller awning and squinted at the rain. Satisfied it was still wet out, she ducked back in again.

"Are you having fun, Camille?" Rosie laughed.

"You bet," I said, my makeup washed away, the money in my fanny pack soaking wet.

Rosie focused her video camera on two young volunteers who were showing off for each other. They sang. "Oh, happy day..." Instantly, all the children joined in. "La, la, la, la, la."

Oh, God, how could they sing now? People were going to think we were nuts.

Jaclyn jumped up, lifted Tiffany into her arms, and started to sway. Tiffany tightened her grip on her sister's neck and hung on for all she was worth. A young mother discreetly gathered her two children close to her as she hurried by.

"Pen," I yelled. "See those people avoiding us? They think Down syndrome's contagious."

The rain let up briefly, and Jo-Layne and some of the children perched on the edge of a large concrete planter, filled with flowers, as they sang. Out of the corner of my eye, I saw a woman nudge the man with her and point at Jo-Layne. Down syndrome, she must have been saying. Tsk, tsk. Her face looked as if she smelled something bad.

I felt my face stiffen. At times like that, I experience the same feelings that every other parent of a handicapped child experiences. I wanted to take the kids home and never let them outside again. Never expose them to contempt. Never risk their feelings or mine. Never put them at society's mercy. But nobody learns anything that way. Nobody learns tolerance or compassion, and nobody learns how to overcome fear. We are part of the world whether we like it or not. Just as important as the next guy. And here we're going to stay.

A group of teenage girls stared openly, then turned their heads and giggled. They were the same age as my volunteers with the same short skirts and long, skinny legs. They had the same braces and eye shadow, yet these girls were so unlike my own teenagers.

I turned to Penny and she nodded. She had seen the girls too. When I linked an arm with Rosie, Penny understood immediately. She grabbed the arm of the volunteer next to her and pulled her over to stand side by side with us. In the rain, we four adults added our voices to the children's chorus. We sang as loudly as we could. "LA, LA, LA, LA, LA." Not knowing my family was their loss.

5 Kyle

❧

*T*eresa understood. "Before my son Kyle was born, I had a different opinion about the handicapped. I didn't hate them, you know that," she said to me. "I just didn't care." She was waiting in my office while Penny went to get Kyle. A small woman with a dancer's posture, she sat quietly and watched the door. With her were her two other children: Kyle's younger sister Kristen, a toddler with blond curls, and his older sister Katie, a composed six-year-old.

Teresa settled down on the floor and pulled her younger daughter onto her lap. She was Puerto Rican, and her husband worked for the FBI on assignment in Puerto Rico, but Kyle was born here in Florida. "He looked s-o-o cute when he was born," Teresa reminisced, smiling at the memory. "He had no hair, no eyelashes, no eyebrows. He was just red and bumpy."

When the doctors told her that his ears were too low, and his head much too large for a child that size, Teresa said that he looked fine to her. When they told her to look at the size of his hands and feet, to see how abnormally big they were, she told them he had beautiful hands and feet. To Teresa there was nothing wrong with them. I didn't see Kyle when he was born, but I am certain he wasn't cute. From the beginning, the doctors knew something was wrong. Kyle was retarded, but they didn't know why. The doctors were stymied at the unusual and unidentified syndrome. Finally, a geneticist was called in. Teresa knew what lay ahead for Kyle in her country. In Puerto Rico, if you had a handicapped child, you put him in a chair, fed him, loved him, and that was it. There were two other retarded people in her family, twins, a boy and a girl. After they were born, their mother put them in a bed. Thirty years later, they are still there, adults the size of six-year olds.

Kyle was eventually diagnosed with monosomy 9p syndrome, a rare chromosomal disorder, so rare that he was one of only ninety-eight known cases in the world. When the geneticist learned that Teresa's husband wanted her to look into alternative arrangements for Kyle, he told her about us.

As Kristen began to fuss, Teresa stood up and held the child in her arms while she swayed back and forth. The little girl popped her thumb in her mouth and closed her eyes. "Not long ago, my husband put it in the best words. He said, 'You know, Camille gave Kyle life, and she gave us back our lives.' He's right; you have."

I hadn't given anybody anything, but Kyle's father was right. Their marriage wouldn't have made it. Many marriages don't survive. The birth of a handicapped child heaps enormous stress and financial burden on a family. The new baby demands time and attention, and that often interferes with the relationship between the parents. They would have been a broken family. So what started as a temporary arrangement became permanent naturally.

Two years earlier, Kyle's family had been transferred to Arizona. Today Teresa was just visiting. Kristen quieted, and Teresa sat back down on the floor cross-legged and laid the child across her lap as she talked. "I don't worry about him. Oh, I miss him. Until the day I die, I'll miss him. I'll miss him for the little boy I dreamed of having, and I'll miss him for the little boy he is. But if I learn I'm going to die tomorrow, I won't worry. I will know he is here."

Teresa was alone when she brought Kyle to live at the foundation. As she said good-bye, I hugged her for a long time. "He's going to miss you, but I'll be here for him," I said, patting her shoulder. "You can go back to your home, to your husband and to your daughters. I will kiss him for you every night. And when he cries, I will hold him."

I also told Teresa children need the truth. Tell Katie about her brother. She would understand. When Teresa arrived home without Kyle, Katie didn't understand. It was three days before she mentioned his name. "Where is my brother?" Katie had sobbed.

Teresa sat down next to her, wrapped her arms around the little girl, and tried to explain. She talked about his differences and the special medical attention he would need,

. . . . — . . . — . . . . . .

and then she told her that Kyle was going to live with a lady
named Camille who would take care of him.

Katie didn't understand. "What is she going to do with
Kyle?"

"She's going to love him for us."

"Is she going to be his mommy?"

"Yes, I guess so."

"Mommy, I miss him," Katie cried.

"Yes, I do too, but we're going to have to learn to handle it."

Katie thought for a minute. "If she is Kyle's mommy, she
is my mommy too." She paused. "You are my mommy, and
she is my . . . my Mama Camille."

Over the next two years, Katie talked of Kyle often. Well-
adjusted and normal in every way, she seemed to have ac-
cepted the fact that he was living with another family. But
her inside didn't match her outside. One weekend, she and
her mother were enjoying a special vacation in San Diego.
It was an exciting trip. Katie had been waiting a long time
to go to Seaworld and see Shamu the killer whale. But, as
they were driving to the aquatic park, Katie began to cry.

"Okay, what's wrong with you now?" Teresa asked, impatient with her daughter's tears.

"I miss my brother," Katie wailed. "I just don't tell you
all the time, but I miss my brother."

Teresa was shocked. "Why are you starting this now? We're
supposed to be having a—"

"I know, Mommy, but I want him to see Shamu."

When Teresa first came here to the foundation, she had

no idea what she was going to do. She was just looking at alternatives, looking for some way to find a solution to all her pain and sorrow. We gave her the only hope she ever had. "I don't know what he has in him," I told her when she first brought Kyle to us. "I cannot promise you anything. But whatever is there, we'll find it. He will be the best he can be. I will care for him, and I will love him, and I will teach him, and I will teach him, and I will teach him."

As she sat in my office and rocked Kristen, she cried angrily, "The doctors told me Kyle would never walk. Kyle would never talk. Kyle would never know who I was. The other day when I came here, he walked over to some photographs hanging on the wall, and he was pointing at the pictures and telling me in his vocabulary who they were. I want to yell at those jerks in that hospital, 'Don't do this to people. Don't leave them without hope.' They should see him. They should see his eyes. He is beautiful."

Teresa hadn't seen Kyle yet that weekend, and this was her last visit before she returned to Arizona. "I believe everybody has one miracle in their life, and—" She stopped abruptly as Kyle came through the door holding Penny's hand. Penny steered him to within three feet of Teresa, let go of his hand, and left the room. Teresa was right. Those doctors should see his eyes. They were beautiful, huge and hazel, and fringed with long, black lashes.

"Hi!" Teresa said quietly, careful to stay where she was, never taking her eyes off him. Kyle stared at her face, but he didn't move a muscle as Teresa finished what she was say-

. . . .

ing. "Yes, I believe everybody has one . . .What? Oh, no!"
The boy didn't move or change expression, but his eyes slowly
filled with tears.

"Penny!" Teresa called, quietly and evenly. She looked at
me, and I nodded. I didn't interfere. I knew she needed to
handle it. She didn't have the chance to make many decisions for her son. "Come get him, I think he is getting upset. Go call Miss Penny, Katie. It's fine, Kyle. Look, Kristen
has come to see you again."

Kyle's eyes shimmered with unshed tears. It hurt my throat
to watch.

"Penny!" Teresa called again. Henry had heard, and he
walked in and knelt at Kyle's side. "What's your problem?"
he asked softly. Kyle didn't move. He just stared at Teresa. I
thought he was frightened, because he didn't remember her.

"Do you want to play?" Henry asked. Kyle didn't answer.

"Do you want to sit down?" Henry asked even more quietly. Kyle just stared at Teresa.

"Want a cookie?" No response.

"Want some juice?" Henry's voice remained soft and or-
dinary.

"Do whatever you need. Don't worry about me," Teresa
said, still kneeling in front of Kyle.

"Want to go get some juice?" Henry asked.

Kyle nodded with the barest of nods, and Henry reached
for the little boy's hand. Teresa never changed position as he
led her son out of the room. When they had gone, she remained on the floor staring after them. There were no tears.

An hour later, it was time for Teresa to leave. I walked her to the playroom to look for her daughters. We found Kyle and Katie sitting on the steps leading into the room. Katie watched the kids play, and Kyle sipped at a glass of juice. They sat side by side, close together, arms touching, not a hint of space between them.

Teresa finished the sentence she had begun in my office as she gave me a big hug good-bye. "I believe everybody gets one miracle in life. You are our miracle, our Mama Camille."

6 *Mike's Office*

Mike stood on one side of a table in one of the examining rooms in his Miami office. I stood quietly across the table from him. With us were the parents of a Down syndrome baby girl, only two weeks old. At first, stunned at the news that they had a handicapped child, they did little more than cry and seek consolation in each other. Now they were looking for hard facts that they could grasp and deal with. They wanted to know exactly what the syndrome is. As they watched Mike, they prepared themselves for his answers.

"You know about chromosomes? Those bits of matter in the nucleus of every cell that contain our genes? The blueprints that determine our characteristics? Sure, you do," Mike said easily. "Well, in a normal cell, there are twenty-two pairs of autosomes, which are regular chromosomes, and two sex chromosomes for a total of forty-six chromosomes. But in Down syndrome, a common form of mental retardation first described by Dr. J. Langdon Down in the 1800s, there is an extra chromosome on the twenty-first pair, making a cell with forty-seven chromosomes rather than forty-six. This causes the genetic disorder, the developmental disorder, we call Down syndrome.

"In ninety-five percent of the people with Down syndrome, trisomy twenty-one is present. When the egg or the sperm is created, it misdivides and produces an extra chromosome. This faulty cell division can also occur after conception or fertilization. Wherever or whenever it happens, in the sperm, the egg, or after fertilization, it results in a cell with forty-seven chromosomes. Remember, for Down syndrome to occur, that extra chromosome must be on the twenty-first pair of chromosomes.

"Two other ways faulty division can occur are translocation and mosaicism. In translocation, there is an extra twenty-first chromosome, but it is translocated, that is, attached to another chromosome. In one-third of these cases, a parent is a carrier. Mosaicism, which occurs only one percent of the time, results in a mixed pattern of chromosomes in the cells, some cells with forty-seven chromosomes, some with forty-six.

"We're still not sure why Down syndrome happens, but we do know some things. It occurs roughly in one out of eight hundred births. It probably doesn't happen because the mother took drugs, or the father drank, but we're not positive about that. We do know it occurs much more frequently in an older mother." His hand rested lightly on the infant's chest as she lay quietly on the table. "If the mother is thirty-five, the risk is one in two hundred. At forty, the

. . . .

risk is one in a hundred. Beyond that, the risk grows as the age increases. There is also greater risk in a very young mother, in a couple where one parent already has a chromosomal disorder, if a couple has a Down child, or a child with another chromosomal abnormality.

"Researchers are also looking at other possible factors: X rays, hormonal problems, immunological problems, viral infections. But at the moment there is no conclusive evidence. The best defense is prenatal screening. Four of the tests being used today are amniocentesis, chorionic villus sampling, ultrasonography, and alpha-fetoprotein. Amniocentesis is a test in which fetal cells from the amniotic fluid surrounding the baby in the uterus are grown in culture. In chorionic villus sampling, placental tissue itself is tested, while ultrasonography is a sound wave test. Alpha-fetoprotein screening examines the level of a protein called alpha-fetoprotein in the mother. Abnormally low levels can point to a defect in the fetus."

"But, Doctor, she looks fine," the mother said. "Is there any chance our doctor is wrong?"

"No," Mike said firmly and flatly. "There are very real characteristics we look for, a profile the newborn will fit if it has Down syndrome." It was natural for the parents to hope the diagnosis was incorrect. Often the characteristics in a newborn are far less noticeable than when the child is older. But it is important for the parents to begin to accept, if they can, the fact that they have a Down syndrome child. Early acceptance is critical because of the many decisions concerning health care and education that must be made.

"Notice the bridge of her nose. See how wide and flat it is?" Mike asked. "See how the nose is smaller? The facial bones aren't fully developed." He traced a path with his finger along the inner corner of the baby's eye. "The eyes are almond shaped, and there's also an extra fold of skin here at the inside corner of her eye. That's called an epicanthic fold." He spoke softly and matter-of-factly as if he were pointing out the characteristics of a flower.

Calm and natural, his speech soothed and stabilized them. We always talk to families this way, and it always helps. "See those tiny white specks in the iris, the colored part of the eye? They're called Brushfield spots. They're also indicative of Down syndrome."

"Can she smile?" the mother asked. "My aunt said these children couldn't smile."

Her husband made a disgusted noise and ran his hand through his hair. "Her aunt is calling us every day. She's making me crazy."

"She means well," the young mother explained with a pained smile. "She pretends she's calling about her arthritis acting up, but I know she's just concerned about the baby. Besides, it does look like the baby's frowning all the time," she said as she pointed to the baby's face.

Mike cradled the infant's head in his hand and glanced up at me. "Camille?"

"This little frown, you mean?" I asked the mother. "That's just because her muscles aren't developed yet. Of course, she can smile. Remember when you were telling Mike how hard it was for her to drink from a bottle? Here's

. . . .

why. Look inside her mouth. Can you see her palate? The roof of her mouth? See how arched and high it is? On some babies it's so pronounced it's almost a U. That's why it's difficult for her to suck. But she'll learn. It'll just take a lot of patience. There are special nipples that will help too. I'll give you the name before you leave."

The mother paid close attention. The father stood behind her with one hand on the examining table and glanced from Mike's face to his daughter's.

"See how the top of her ear is level with her eye?" Mike asked, then pointed to the mother's ear. "On you and me, the top of our ear is above the level of our eye." Then, using only the baby's hands, he lifted the infant a few inches off the table. "See how her head falls back? Her neck cannot support the weight, and at this age in a normal child, her neck should be able to. She has a pretty good grip though. Some Down babies would let go completely."

The couple exchanged glances, pleased at the good news while Mike unfastened the baby's jumpsuit. "They said she had a hernia. Would you check?" the father asked.

"Frequently, the umbilicus protrudes," Mike said as he examined the baby's abdomen and groin. "Yes, probably an inguinal hernia, not at all uncommon. Don't worry." He held the baby's hand and spread her fingers wide. She screamed at the intrusion. "Shorter fingers, see?"

Tears filled the father's eyes, but Mike continued, knowing the man would be embarrassed if he paused. "Did you know Down children have a different fingerprint pattern, different lines and whorls? And yet, within the syndrome, they each have distinct fingerprints of their own."

I pointed to the baby's foot. "You'll often see a large distance between their big toe and their other toes. That's why some Down children walk the way they do. They use the big toe for balance, and then they roll their foot."

"Can she hear?" the mother asked, her eyes intent on the baby.

Mike clapped his hands behind the baby's head, and the infant jumped and threw her arms out reflexively. Her parents laughed, relieved. Mike dangled his arms at his sides. "See how far down the side of my body my arms hang? Down children have shorter arms and shorter legs." As he refastened the baby's clothing, his voice softened, and he peered into the mother's face. "You okay?"

She nodded. My heart went out to her. "Do you understand a little more now?" She nodded again, her nose red. Both she and her husband were calmer and more relaxed.

"The doctor told you about Camille's foundation, right?" Mike asked kindly. "Come into my office. She can give you some information to take with you. She'll make you feel better. Besides, she's got all kinds of stuff: fact sheets, articles from journals, diet and behavior tips, everything you can think of." We had been with this couple for over an hour, but he didn't rush them. He understood their need for information.

As we sat there in Mike's office, the father glanced worriedly at his wife as he asked, "Dr. Geraldi, we've been hearing about all kinds of medical problems that develop later on. We understand Judith has one hole in her heart that requires surgery. What else can we expect?"

"There are a variety of problems associated with Down syndrome. Probably forty percent of these children have heart defects, so you're not alone. Digestive problems and bowel obstructions are other problems we see a lot of. There are respiratory infections, hearing difficulties, eye problems, and other things, but right now she has none of these that I can see. So don't look for trouble. We'll keep an eye out and take them as they come. All right?"

"Doctor, was there something we should have done differently before she was born? We feel like it's our fault," the father asked, hesitatingly. "The mental re-retardation? How bad is it?"

"I don't know. We won't know for a little while. We'll test her now, and then we'll be able to give you a better estimate of her capabilities in a month or so. But, as many people will tell you, *she will be more like other children than unlike them*," Mike replied.

I handed them a folder filled with information and held the mother's gaze. "Remember that. She will be more like other children than unlike them. She'll just be on a different timetable. And it's not your fault. It's important to remember that too."

We talked for a few more minutes, and as the couple started to leave, the mother turned back impulsively and hugged Mike and me. As Mike patted her back and smiled at the husband over her shoulder, Mike said, "You'll see, this baby will be the light of your life."

As we walked them to the reception area, Mike offered some more encouragement. "There are many things you can do to help your child reach her full potential." He ticked them off on his fingers, "Infant stimulation, environment, interaction, exercise, and early intervention."

In one office visit, often it wasn't prudent or possible to explain all the traits of Down syndrome. There are, however, over fifty characteristics that make up the Down syndrome profile. In addition to the ones Mike described, there are Spock-shaped ears with thinner ear cartilage than normal; brachycephaly, a larger head, flatter in the back; and the simian crease, an unpleasant phrase that describes a line that runs across the palm of the hand. The tongue is thick and difficult to control. In many of these children, the poor muscle tone combines with some hearing difficulty to create a special challenge for speech therapists. Down syndrome children and adults seem to speak in telegrams. They either can't hear or don't grasp the small words, the prepositions and conjunctions that smooth our language and make the path to understanding easier to follow and quicker to learn. Much work has been done in this area, though, and there is a great deal of literature available.

More examples of the medical complaints include ear ailments, myopia (nearsightedness), and hypothyroidism (insufficient thyroid hormones) in adults. Almost all Down syndrome children have some problem in the physical makeup of their ears that requires careful, attentive medical treatment. Frequent eye examinations are important. Nearsightedness is not a rare complaint. Hypothyroidism, if monitored, can be corrected with medication. All of these problems must be watched to avoid complications.

There are many things parents can do to offset or minimize the fact that Down syndrome children usually sit up, stand, walk, and toilet train more slowly than other children. The key is early intervention. Along with social workers, special teachers, and physical, occupational, and speech therapists, it takes one-on-one training and extra assistance for developmentally delayed children. The earlier the training begins, the better—under the age of five is ideal. Training takes place either at home with the therapist or teacher or at a center or school, or at a combination of the two.

Experts emphasize that the structure and content of early intervention techniques are of primary importance. Individual educational programs are drawn up to set goals and monitor progress in areas such as speech and fine and gross motor skills. Infants, like adults, need to interact with their world. They must be able to reach for something and then grab it. As they develop, they must learn what an object is and what it does. Babies need to master physical actions: lift and turn their heads, roll over, sit up, learn hand-eye coordination and depth perception.

Stimulation means literally waking the brain, firing the neurons that set in place the paths and avenues of more complex thought. A parent or teacher must stir the fire until it sparks, catches, and finally leaps to life. Ideally, this should begin at birth. With exercise, sensory awareness, and language, parents and teachers can expand the senses of an infant in many fun ways. (See Appendix B, Stimulation Techniques.) Most important, the underlying philosophy of early intervention should be the philosophy of everyone who interacts on a regular basis with that baby. The child should grow up in a stimulating, happy, sound-filled, tactile environment, peopled with those who care.

It also makes financial sense to begin education at an early age in order to help a child live a more independent, perhaps self-supporting life. Although not the paramount reason for early intervention, it is a valid, important argument for it. As Mike said, there are many things that can be done and learned to add to the quality of the child's life. Along with everything else he mentioned, there are computer speech programs, job training programs, and additional computer programs for vision and hearing to help Down syndrome children express the thoughts they cannot say. Mainstreaming them in regular schools and teaching them independent living skills are also options. The list is long, hopeful, and invaluable.

Given more time, Mike would certainly have told them to share the diagnosis and their feelings. (See Appendix A, Family Feelings.) He would have advised them to tell their family and friends, put a note in the birth announcement, or make a telephone call. This builds a support network for the family and makes it easier to face others after the birth. It will also help avoid unintentionally hurtful remarks from those who don't know.

*I*t was still early as Mike and I headed for Baptist Hospital. It had rained, and some of the side streets were flooded, so he took a circuitous route he knew like the back of his hand. He drove a doctor's car, a shiny black Mercedes, big and immaculate, not a speck of dust in the interior. On this slick, sleek car, the license frame read ASK ME ABOUT DOWN SYNROME. On the seat beside him was a black mace gun to match. The car gave you a good idea of what he did for a living, while the mace gun told you a lot about the unwelcome atmosphere in Miami.

The nurse at the nurse's station nodded. "Good to see you, Dr. Geraldi. Camille, how are you?"

Mike smiled and exchanged brief pleasantries, but his step was brisk and eager as he turned and pushed open the door to his patient's room. He said hello to the mother and father, washed his hands at the sink, and turned to take the well-wrapped infant from his father. "How is he?"

Ten minutes later, almost finished with the examination, Mike placed his thumbs near the baby's fingers, waited for him to grasp them, and then tried to lift him four or five inches off the bed. The baby's grip loosened quickly, and his head lolled back on his neck. But Mike didn't look concerned. After all, this child did not have Adelle's Down syndrome, or Kyle's rare monosomy 9p syndrome, or Jo-Layne's enlarged heart, or cystic fibrosis, or spina bifida, or any one of the dozens and dozens of other heartaches. These parents were blessed. This child was normal.

Five minutes later, the routine, cursory exam was over,

and the baby was rewrapped and sleeping in his father's arms. "Remember, call me if you have any questions, any at all. Keep him warm, make sure anyone who touches him washes their hands first. That's important. If they have a cold or a touch of something, keep them away. They can see him another time. I'll see you in two weeks."

Mike's hair was down today, long enough to bounce on his collar like a hippie's as he led me toward the elevator. One more baby to check.

I waited by the door in the tiny anteroom as Mike met with the parents and examined the baby. This newborn, only one day old, hung on tight, his neck stiff and strong, when Mike lifted him with his thumbs. "Oh my goodness," he said with a delighted smile and a look at the mother to see if she was noticing her baby's prowess. She was answering the phone, but grinned and nodded back.

As the baby started to cry, he turned it over and held the infant, stomach down, on his hand. "Puts pressure on the diaphragm if you do this. See? It's harder to cry in this position," he said. He ran his fingers down either side of the baby's spine, listened to his chest, and checked the umbilical cord while the baby screamed his head off. "Well, it's supposed to be harder for them to cry in this position." He laughed at himself, chagrined.

When he finished the examination, the mother was still on the phone. So he wrapped the baby up and stood there holding him while she tried to get rid of her caller. The baby settled down, and Mike smiled. He wasn't impatient, wasn't

. . . .

angry. The tail of the blanket worked its way loose as he jiggled the baby. He didn't notice. His body language said, there's no rush. It did not say, my wife is going to kill me if I don't hurry up. "Don't hesitate to call," he said softly, depositing the baby in its mother's arms. "Don't hesitate." He must have said that a thousand times a day.

In our hectic world, he was an oasis for me, a calm and sane place. Definitely an unusual man, though. Today he wore an upscale biker's belt covered with metal studs, a gold neck chain, and designer glasses. On the staffs of Miami's major hospitals where the doctor's uniform of the day is a conservative gray suit, this morning Mike's shirt was covered with stars and half moons, a magician's costume more than a doctor's uniform.

When I'm not with him, and he's talking one-on-one to a client, or lecturing before a group, Mike is in charge. His voice carries. His posture is relaxed and expansive. He seems bigger. But when we're together, my personality takes up a lot of room, and Mike is quieter, more comfortable talking about me than himself. But, my word, can he say some strange things!

"I believe Camille lived before," he told a reporter. He just said it as naturally as if he had said I lived in Peoria. I didn't believe it until I read the paper the next day. He told the same reporter that I could tell if a child was sick by his or her smell. It was true, but can you imagine how that looked in print? It sounded like I went around sniffing the children.

7 *Joelle*

Henry is a young man on my staff. He and I have a particular connection.

In khaki shorts and a turquoise golf shirt, a small gold earring in his left ear, Henry sat quietly in an easy chair in the living room while the rest of the house got ready for dinner. Skinny and the color of butterscotch syrup, Henry is the half-Polish, half-Japanese husband of Penny, our British beatnik. He wears his hair long in back, cropped short around his ears. A quiet man who talks very slowly and acts older than his twenty-seven years, Henry moves without fuss or noise. He just seems to appear in a room. While he works at the foundation, he is studying to become a doctor.

Before his marriage to Penny and his job at the foundation, Henry had been dating a woman I'll call Diane. They dated for a while, but when the relationship didn't work out, the couple drifted apart. Months later, Diane's dad called Henry. During the startling conversation, Henry discovered that he was a father. Diane had given birth to a little girl. By the end of the phone call, Henry learned the child had Down syndrome. He quickly decided what he wanted to do, and tried to explain to Diane's father.

"Marriage is only if she wants to, because it's useless to get married for a kid. Down the road, you break up and the kid is the one who pays. I'd be willing to quit school, though, because the child comes first. I'll get a full-time job, go in the military, whatever I need to do. That baby is my responsibility."

When he saw Diane the next day, she made it immediately clear that she was going to put the baby up for adoption. Trying to be realistic, Henry didn't fight her. He knew that no matter what he did, there was no way he could raise that baby by himself. No matter how many resources he pulled together, he wouldn't be able to make it.

Diane decided not to see the baby. It would only make it harder, she told her family. I don't know if she was overwrought or overwhelmed. Who can ever say how another person really feels? Henry went to see the baby, though. He went before he signed the papers releasing his rights as a father, and he kept right on going.

Seriously ill with lung problems and a gravely underdeveloped heart, the baby was transferred to pediatric intensive care at Sacred Heart Hospital in Pensacola. When doctors discovered the extent of her heart problems, she was prepared for another transfer, this time to a hospital in Miami. While she was still in Pensacola, Henry and his mother, a loving moral support through it all, drove there every other night to see her. Even though the infant was very ill, they were still able to hold and feed her. It probably was no surprise to Henry's mom that her son was falling in love with his daughter.

Because the baby had Down syndrome and so many other serious medical problems, the attorney hired by Diane was unable to find an adoptive family for the infant. When the lawyer asked Henry if he wanted to take custody of the baby, he said yes. He was willing to be a single parent at twenty-three. I'm sure that didn't surprise his mother either.

The night before he was to sign the adoption papers, knowing it was the last night he would be going out for a while, Henry celebrated. At seven the next morning, the attorney called him again. She had found a family to adopt the baby.

Angry and hurt at being bounced back and forth, Henry never had the opportunity to sign the adoption papers. He had no say in the arrangements. It was definite. His daughter was going to live with another family. Powerless, but not satisfied with the attorney's decision, Henry wanted to see this family for himself. The adoptive mother had already told the attorney Henry could contact her. Her name was Camille Geraldi.

In August, while I was overseeing the last session of the summer camp at our cabin in North Carolina, I received a telephone call from an attorney who had been referred to me by Health and Rehabilitative Services. A critically ill

. . . .

Down syndrome baby had been born at Sacred Heart Hospital, and the mother had given it up for adoption. Would I take it? Of course, I would.

Two weeks later, on August 24, 1990, the baby was flown by air ambulance from Sacred Heart Hospital to Miami. A medical transport team traveled with her to monitor her progress and provide care in case, God forbid, something happened. It was a difficult time, trying to arrange the transfer, straighten out Medicaid, and get the legal papers ready. I was so excited though, it didn't matter. A new baby, and a girl at that!

I already knew something about the baby's background, so I wasn't surprised when Henry called. From then on, I kept him informed at every turn. I told him up front we were going to have our hands full, because she was in such bad shape.

I named her carefully. She was going to need divine providence for the months ahead. Because Jo-Layne and Adelle had been so sick and still survived, I thought if I combined their names, it would bring her special luck. I named her Joelle.

During the first week, to determine the extent of Joelle's heart problems, Dr. Lee Ann Pearce performed a cardiac catheterization. The physician threaded a tiny narrow, plastic tube through an artery into Joelle's heart and injected a dye into the tube. It was a tricky procedure that the infant tolerated poorly. After it was over, I wrote in her chart at the foundation: "Barely in existence. Bad pathology."

Although she was underweight and on a heart monitor, Joelle was able to go home with us on September 4. Within days, Henry came down to see the baby and to meet us. He ended up spending four days at the foundation. He fit in well. When he went back home, I told Mike, "You mark my words, he'll be back."

I was right. He called me first. I smiled to myself at his embarrassment. He hurried his words as if to get the sentence over with, nervous at his own boldness.

"Camille, I went home and thought about it, and I—I wonder if you and Mike would let me live at the foundation and work there while I go to school. It was made for me, me wanting to be a doctor and all, and I've already worked with handicapped kids."

"Can you handle this kind of work?" I asked him. "It's not easy." Most people couldn't.

"The way Christopher looked, you know, with his big head and all, that kind of threw me in the beginning, but other than that, I can handle it. I can handle anything, except for Joelle."

I agreed, and Henry moved in right away. It was good for him. He needed our support. Joelle was a very difficult and fragile baby. Feeding her was awful. Her respirations were so rapid that she couldn't hold her breath long enough to swallow her formula. She vomited at least once a day. We had to keep her upright all the time. But she was beautiful. She looked like a little angel.

Within a month, Joelle was vomiting at every feeding and

had to be readmitted to the hospital. But, even at three months, she was a fighter, and before long, she was home again for a few weeks. By Thanksgiving, she had been in and out of the hospital again. Still, we were thankful to have her home for the holiday. Thirty-six hours later, she had seizures, and we rushed her back to the hospital.

During that hospitalization, there were many problems. Joelle endured being poked and prodded as long as she could, until finally she couldn't stand it anymore. She wouldn't let anyone hold her, not even me. But on January 4, she swung around again. She let me hold her. I swore that child had 965 lives.

I also had Kellie-Ann in the hospital, upstairs on 6B for open-heart surgery. When one of the children is in the hospital, everything else in my life stops. It has to. In a large, crowded hospital, it's very difficult to get special, individual care from the already overworked nursing staff. I put everything on hold and I spent ten hours a day at that hospital caring for those two children. There was no time for anything else, not even a minute to sit down and check in with myself to see how *I* was doing.

Joelle was off antibiotics by January 18 and due to go home the next day. Late that afternoon, one of her doctors called me. Her condition had nosedived, and she had been rushed to intensive care. The possible diagnosis was a rampant, systemwide infection—sepsis.

"Sepsis?" I asked. "No way, we just stopped all antibiotics yesterday. I totally disagree." What were they thinking? I asked myself. She might have had infections, but this plummet in her condition was from her heart, I was sure. She needed oxygen. Henry always complained that the people who worked in most hospitals didn't treat our children the way they treated the other kids. They didn't pay enough attention to them, because they were retarded or because they were Medicaid patients. The care was different, however, for patients with private insurance. I sometimes wondered if he wasn't right.

All through January, Joelle struggled back, fighting valiantly. On Thursday, February 7, they removed the airway tubing. It was one more long and painful procedure. Joelle smiled halfway through the two and a half hour ordeal. After it was over, I knew we were in for a tough go. She was either coming back to stay, or, when she smiled, she had seen those Pearly Gates.

At that point, Henry got scared. He saw Joelle one night when she was in ICU, and she looked bad. She was getting so many drugs by then that she didn't even resemble herself, and she was in a lot of pain. He didn't know what to think. That was the first time Henry prayed that his daughter would die, just to end her suffering.

Saturday morning before the sun was up, an intensive care nurse called. Joelle's breathing had worsened. "It's very slow and labored, Camille." Over those months, I had received a lot of other calls about Joelle. That time though, I knew. But just in case I was wrong, I didn't want to alarm Henry, not just yet. I wanted to wait and see Joelle myself, before I called him. So Mike and I hurried to the hospital by ourselves, without saying anything. We were there in less than ten minutes. Later, when I had time to think, I was sorry I had made that decision.

Like my tough Jo-Layne, throughout her life, Joelle had grit. Only six months old, Joelle had struggled through crisis after crisis. But at sunrise that morning, in whisper-quiet dignity, with a soft, then softer breath, Joelle died.

I called Henry from the hospital. Eunice was working with him, and, as soon as she saw his face, she knew what had happened. He had a syringe in his hand, and he threw it across the desk. Within minutes, he met us at the hospital as we were taking her body to the undertaker. She was so little, I didn't want to leave her in the hospital morgue.

It was a difficult time for all of us. I don't think Henry and I said a dozen words to each other. We couldn't. I didn't ask him how he was feeling, and he didn't ask me. It was just too hard. We reminded each other too much of the baby we had lost.

We publish a newsletter at the foundation, and in the March issue, I wrote: "Her soul is at peace, the peace we all deserve when we work so hard to do our best each and every day."

A year later, Henry still had trouble talking about Joelle. So did I. We were sitting outside in the backyard one day watching Karley and some of the other young children play, and he began to open up.

"When I first saw her after she was born, she looked like

a little doll. She was so small when I held her that her feet were at my fingertips, and her head was at my elbow." He bent his arm gently as if cradling her.

"Remember that red hair she had in the beginning? And those hazel eyes? Or were they blue? It's hard to remember back that far. I remember when I first saw her, I thought she looked like her mother. When I think of her now, I just see her in the hospital at the end with all those tubes in her.

"On her birthday, I was a real bear. I wasn't sociable and I didn't want to do anything. I had a real short fuse that day." His voice was barely audible, and he made no attempt to wipe the tears off his cheeks. "I wonder what she would look like. I look at these kids, and I wonder how tall she would be. I wonder . . ."

He sat up straight, took a deep breath, and planted his hands on his knees. "I think she was put here on purpose. I always wanted to go to medical school, and I really didn't have the grades. I think that she was a way of getting me here, into this environment. I'm doing a lot better in school now. I don't go out and drink anymore. I know Joelle was put here to help me get my life straightened out."

He glanced up at a noise he had heard. The older children must have just come home from school. You could hear them carrying on. Yells and shouts. Lots of laughs and hollering. One of the adults called Henry's name, and he grinned sad and sweet. "The one thing that helped me through all that was Karley. She's the one I'm closest with. When Karley was asleep, I used to talk to her about Joelle."

As Henry talked, I thought of him at the dining room table with Karley. Their heads touched as they shared a bowl of ice cream. Henry spooned one spoonful for Karley, one for himself, one for Karley, one for himself.

My grieving was different than Henry's. I am normally an organized and focused person. I had learned through the years that it is important to keep my feelings carefully tucked away so that I could always deal clearly and matter-of-factly with the children's illnesses and emergencies. I have trained my staff to do the same.

But when Joelle died, I was absolutely unprepared for the grief and pain I felt. I couldn't handle it. "Mike, I can't stand this. No more newborns. Let's stop for a while. Let's stop." I had decided not to adopt any more babies. It was emotionally too hard.

After that, life was emptier for us, but we went on. At least, we went through the motions. What else were we going to do? Looking back on it, I wasn't myself. Mike had always talked about the beginning of our relationship and how difficult it was to get close to me. I think I tried to make my life that way again, when I was in control of my emotions. I recreated an ordered world filled with people whose temperaments didn't rock the boat or disrupt the system. Belligerent and strong-willed employees learned the hard way that access to that world was not easy.

I was trying to rebuild the world I had created when I started the foundation, an orderly environment, structured and secure, where my nails were carefully manicured and my hair was perfectly combed, where all the cans in the kitchen cupboard faced front and where my children were always safe. But the effort was exhausting. I was always tired.

We used to have a cook, but Mike and I needed to get away once in a while, so, to afford that, I let the cook go. Now I cook every night for thirty-five people. With the money we paid the cook, Mike and I rent a little apartment on the beach where two nights a month I sleep for fifteen hours at a time. Without that time alone, just the two of us, we couldn't survive. Oh, the babies come with me, but no one else. None of the other children. Only two or three of the staff, and Renae and Jaclyn, of course. But no one else.

8 *Ada*

Bill took two photos of Courtney only seconds apart. In the first, the camera captured her full face, nose flat, eyes oddly shaped. A second later, he snapped her picture again. She had moved slightly, and now the camera revealed another Courtney —a three-quarter face. The wide bridge of her nose was gone. Her nose turned up, pert and cute. Her eyes were a beautiful shape and size. The Down syndrome had disappeared. She looked normal.

There are some teachers and social workers who tell distraught parents that their Down syndrome child could grow up to be normal. That isn't true. No matter how many times the camera fooled us, Courtney would never be normal. She was loving and caring and very special, but she was not normal, and she was never going to be.

Ada had wanted her son Albert to be born normal. But Albert was born with Down syndrome. Shortly after the delivery, as Ada lay in her hospital bed trying to come to grips with what had happened, her doctor walked in. In the room's deafening quiet, his words dropped like stones. Her son would never lift his head. He would never speak or walk. Be brave, be strong, the doctor said. There was more. Her husband was threatening to kill himself. There she was, flat on her back, a mother with an eleven-year-old at home, with her own mother and sisters downstairs in the waiting room hysterically crying, a suicidal husband in the hall, and her newborn with Down syndrome. And her doctor told her she was supposed to be strong.

Ada and her husband took Albert home, and somehow life went on. Her son Tommy went to school, and her husband went back to work, while Ada sat at home in desperation and cried. For two weeks, she stayed in bed and wept until a worried neighbor telephoned her own pediatrician to see if he could help. At that point, I knew fate had stepped in. The pediatrician's name was Dr. Geraldi.

Later that day, Ada was still in bed when I called her. I explained who I was and told her my experiences with Down syndrome. "I know you see everything as black and white," I said calmly.

"Hm-hmm," Ada replied through her tears, trying to speak. "They say my son will never ride a bike."

"Baloney! Who says he won't ride a bike?" I cried. "Who told you that? Your son is going to be whatever you make of him."

"M-m-m," Ada answered, her words caught in her throat.

"Right now you think this is the end of your life, don't you?" I asked. "Well, it isn't. It's just the beginning."

. . . .

Ada could not afford the physical therapists and other spe-
cialists Albert needed, so she turned to the foundation for
help. The staff and I taught her the exercises to strengthen
Albert's muscles and improve his balance and coordination.
She did them faithfully, 150 times each day. Every two weeks,
I taught her new ones; then she went back to Albert and
practiced those exercises 150 times a day. She stayed home
that first year and concentrated all her efforts on him. He
walked at fourteen months.

When Albert was four, his father left them. I wasn't surprised.

Albert is five now, and Ada's seventy-six-year-old mother
cares for him while Ada works. Albert's grandmother has
always said he is normal. When Ada tries to tell her the truth,
his grandmother weeps. "He's not retarded. He's not retarded." Ada finally gave up trying.

"My son has changed all our lives," Ada said one afternoon. "I'm different. I look at things differently. How the
house looks, what material things I have is not so important
anymore. I see it in my clients at work too. The ones with
handicapped children are like me. They are different. My
other clients are not. They talk about their problems with
the husband or with the house. I say to them, be thankful
every day for what you have. My son thinks he's a king, because we treat him like one. After Albert was born, when I
was lying in bed crying, I hadn't been looking for help.
I had been looking for hope. That's what you gave me,
Camille—hope."

. . . .

"It's more than hope," I said. "You've gained confidence in yourself. You know you can handle this." Ada didn't need me the way she used to. She had learned how to do things for herself, how to take care of her son, where to go to solve a problem, and what agencies to call for help. She could stand on her own, and she could fight the world.

"You are right. I can handle it. Oh, I know Albert is not normal, but I also know he's just another child, another human being. And I'm going to give it the best I can. He's great. And guess what happened at school?" she said, beaming with pride. "He was just suspended for two days."

All the parents love to tell me the newest stories about their kids, bragging about their pranks and misadventures. They tell their story with half smiles, knowing I'll laugh and shake my head and delight with them in the normalcy of their kid being just a kid.

The day Albert was born, his brother, Tommy, came to the hospital to visit him. It frightened Tommy to see his grandmother and aunts crying in the waiting room. He wondered if something had happened to his mom. When he saw that Ada was fine, he was confused. "Why is everybody crying?"

"Because the baby is sick, Tommy," Ada replied.

"No, I just saw him, Mom," he cried excitedly. "In the nursery. Go see him. He's fine!"

"No," Ada said gently. "He might look fine now, but he's not. He has Down syndrome."

Tommy frowned. "What is that?"

Ada carefully explained everything to her son. She was

worried about his reaction, but she wanted to be honest. She told him that the baby was healthy, but he would be slower than the other children, and he would look different than they did.

But this was a kid with his priorities straight. "Is that all?" he asked.

9 *The Easter Bunny*

*M*y kids waited on blankets spread out under the trees in the backyard with the staff. I had even recruited Rick from the night shift to help. We were going to need it. We were celebrating outdoors because I had lived through too many messy Easter mornings. We had lined the basket earlier with yellow Easter grass and filled it with hard-boiled eggs we dyed the previous night, and candy, a rare treat. As soon as the kids spied Easter Bunny Mike carrying candy in a laundry basket, they went crazy.

I stayed in the background supervising and videotaping. The staff and volunteers ran around and grabbed the kids so they wouldn't trample Mike. Later on, I saw myself on the videotape. Captain Camille, in the flesh. Talk about the kids getting a little loud!

I watched Courtney thrust a piece of candy covered with grass into her mouth. Before anyone could grab it away from her, I yelled. It sounded as if I had just hit the button on my megaphone. "Take that grass out of her mouth!"

I laughed when Champ snatched a chocolate-covered marshmallow bunny from the basket and danced away, tearing at the wrapper. In seconds, he had chocolate on his shirt, his face, his hands, his pants. He had chocolate on his chocolate. "M-m-m!" was all he said.

"Say thank you, Champie," someone yelled.

"M-m-m," was as close as he got.

Mike set the basket of candy on a blanket, and the kids surrounded it instantly. Kyle and some of the other smarter ones plopped down next to it and staked their claim. I saw Kyle's chin hanging over the edge of the basket, all eyes as everyone reached around him and grabbed the candy. Kyle didn't understand.

"Penny, give some to Kyle," I hollered. I wanted to be everywhere at once.

Jaclyn, with Christopher in her lap, laughed and yelled at one of her friends while she stuck a piece of marshmallow in Christopher's mouth. He shuddered as if it were castor oil and shook his head at the taste. He didn't want any part of it.

And Jo-Layne? My Jo-Layne was in hog heaven. She sat cross-legged on the grass, with a foot-high chocolate bunny she had grabbed out of the basket. Bending over, she planted her mouth on the bunny's ears and ate her heart out.

"Who gave that to her?" I cried, laughing hysterically as I watched my daughter eat. "Who wouldn't love chocolate? That's my favorite food."

It didn't matter to Jo-Layne how envious I was. She never even glanced at me.

"Mom, Mariah doesn't like it," Renae hollered. She pointed to Mariah who was making a face and crying.

When Mariah was only a few days old, her Haitian parents abandoned her at a county hospital. Born with Down syndrome and a grave blood disorder, Mariah was very ill and on her own in the world. Comatose, unresponsive to anything, she lay in that hospital bed for six months, existing in a world of minimal care and little affection.

When I received a request from the hospital to visit her, I went right away. The doctors asked me to try and stimulate her, see if I could get some kind of response. I was unsuccessful. As I walked out of that cold, overcrowded building, I was certain that Mariah was going to live out her life there. I couldn't let that happen, so I decided to talk to Mike.

Mike hadn't made a fuss when we adopted Darlene, because she was so light-skinned. He knew she would easily fit in with our family. He wasn't prejudiced, just worried about how other people would treat her. But Mariah was the first dark-skinned child that I had wanted to adopt. My husband didn't approve.

"I don't think it's wise, that's all," he explained. "You always have to look at the repercussions on the child, Camille."

I couldn't leave her in that hospital, so I made plans to bring her home. Mike didn't even know. When I thought about it later, I was astonished at myself. That night when he came home from work, I was sitting in a chair with the new infant on my lap. Mike stopped and stared at us, but I just smiled, with my heart in my throat, and tried to sound a lot more confident than I felt. "Well, this is your black child, Mariah."

At first, he didn't say anything. I was so worried. He had always let me do anything I wanted, but he was quiet for so long that I thought I had finally gone too far. Then I realized that he was crying.

"Well, we're on a roll," he said with a watery laugh. "But where did you get the name Mariah?"

I laughed with such relief. "I named her after the Marion nuns I used to volunteer with when I was a kid." I held Mariah out to him. "You see, this is what I've worked for all my life."

But as the days passed, no matter how hard I tried, I couldn't get Mariah to respond to anything. I used all the tricks I knew, but nothing had any effect on her. I carefully held her in front of me and moved her through the air like a little airplane. I stuck her in an infant seat and sat her down in the middle of whatever was going on. We talked to her and laughed as if she was awake, curious, and aware. I encouraged the other children to play and yell and carry on around her. Anything to stimulate her! I blared the radio. We turned the television set up. Champ and Karley stumbled over her, the dog sniffed her foot, and all the children hugged her and gave her kisses. Yet in the midst of all the laughter and noise, Mariah never moved.

A month later, there was still no change. I clapped and turned her when I turned the other children. I tube-fed her and massaged the muscles in her arms and legs with strong, even strokes. I held her on my lap, facing out, so she could "see" the world. And I chattered and sang to her all the time with lots of inflection in my voice. Out of habit, I used great, oversized gestures. But nothing helped. She just lay there, wherever I put her, never moving. Her eyes never opened.

One night she was lying on the changing table, while I washed her face and talked to Jaclyn across the room. As I reached for the towel on the back of the table, I sensed a movement out of the corner of my eye. I froze. When I looked down, Mariah was in the same position, still as a stone. Nothing had changed. I was seeing things.

I reached again for the towel. At the edge of my vision, I saw something. I was certain. "Mariah, can you hear me?" I asked, trying to keep my voice calm. "Can you hear Mommy?"

I thought she moved her foot.

"Mariah! Mommy's talking to you. Can you hear me?" She moved her foot.

I waited for a moment without saying anything. She didn't twitch a muscle.

"Mariah Geraldi, you little devil, if you can hear me, you'd better let me know, or . . ."

She moved her foot.

"Jaclyn, go get your father. Quick!"

When Mike hurried into the room, he checked for himself.

"It's Daddy, Mariah. Can you open your eyes for Daddy?"

She lay there, unmoving.

"Mariah? Mariah?" I pleaded with tears in my eyes. "Show your daddy your mommy's not crazy."

She moved her foot.

"Well, I'll be darned," Mike said, and a grin spread across his face like the sun.

At first, Mariah responded only to me and to the sound of my voice. But as the weeks went on, she recognized other voices, reacting more and more each day. Within six weeks, she was awake and fully responsive. Within a year, she was trying to crawl. At two, she walked.

By the time she was five, she had skin as smooth and shiny as the chocolate on a Mounds bar and a mind of her own. She loved and always wore a chartreuse-and-black bathing suit. When it grew too small, she refused to give it up. Trotting around in that old, skintight suit, her stomach pooched out in front, she looked as if she had swallowed a bowling ball.

We discovered she was high functioning, but, wow, was she a handful! God gave her beautiful skin and lovely hair to make up for her long, jutting boxer's chin. I braided her hair in corn rows and strung colored beads on the ends. That helped. But she still looked like she wanted to punch you in the mouth.

Mariah was different from the other children too. They were used to visitors coming and going in our home, and it never bothered them. Not Mariah. Whenever she spotted new people in the house, she narrowed her eyes and watched them, as if she believed they were planning to steal the silver.

"Mom, I said Mariah doesn't like this Easter candy," Renae cried.

I tried to film everything, but I wasn't used to the darned camera. "Renae, give her a yellow chick. I can't . . ." I saw something out of the corner of my eye. "He just put that whole bunny in his mouth."

Leanne watched the children demolish the candy as she edged closer and closer to the basket. When she leaned over one of the kid's heads to look inside, Bill realized what she was waiting for.

"The adults! Camille, the adults!" he yelled and reached into the basket for their candy. He didn't want one of the kids to grab the big chocolate bunnies reserved for Joanne and Leanne and the other adults.

"Uh-oh," he said as he counted the bunnies in his hands. "Here, Leanne. Joanne, here's yours." We were one short. He glanced at Jo-Layne.

Uh-oh was right. Jo-Layne didn't care how many bunnies they were short. She didn't care if they starved. She had eaten down to the rabbit's eyebrows on some unlucky adult's bunny, and as far as she was concerned, she owned it.

"No!" Champ yelled at Renae. I swung the camera around toward the sound of his voice. He stood rigid and held his hand out.

"Wait a minute," she ordered. All she was trying to do

was take the wrapper off his candy. Karley hung over her shoulder, watching, her candy already unwrapped.

I knew what she was about to do. "Bite, Karley, bite. Don't put that whole thing in your mouth at once."

Tiffany shoved pink marshmallow rabbits into her mouth as fast as she could lift her arm, doing a fairly good job for someone with half her teeth missing. Matthew, covered in chocolate, rubbed his hands together like the candy was a bar of soap.

There was chocolate everywhere. On their faces, their clothes, in their hair, all over the blankets. Adelle was my only fastidious child. Every time she discovered some melted candy on her hand, she carefully wiped it off on Wendy's arm. Wendy, one of my Down syndrome adults, busy eating, never noticed.

Two Girl Scout volunteers stood off to the side and watched. Not a muscle in their young bodies moved. Their uniforms were spotless. They weren't about to get in this mess.

"Now Darlene doesn't like hers," Renae cried. "How come some of them like it and some of them hate . . ."

"Christopher, hold your head up."

"Renae, that's because it's not melted or mangled enough. Isn't it, Dar?" Penny asked, laughing.

I was sure Kyle had not moved from the basket. He stretched his hand out for more candy, but his mouth was so full he couldn't chew or swallow. Renae reached down and held on to his hands until he had his mouth under control. Across from him, Mariah wolfed down yellow chicks as fast as she could swallow.

Jo-Layne was finally full or sick or both, and she reached out for me to pick her up. But I had my hands full with the camera. "Hold on to Mommy's leg," I told her. "That will have to do until I can pick you up."

Mike scooped her up for me and held her while he watched the others. "Wave to Bill," he coaxed. When she didn't respond, he blew gently into her face to get her attention. "Wave to Bill." Mike patted her back and smiled to himself at the commotion in front of him.

"This was a nice Easter, Cooch."

10 *Rachael, Meredith, and Carmelo*

✿

I was still tired a week later, but the day was almost over. The only thing left on my schedule was Rachael's physical therapy session. Rachael is a sixteen-year-old girl with Down syndrome and cerebral palsy who lives at the foundation in respite care. Cerebral palsy, a crippling disorder, results from damage to the central nervous system. Muscles always twitching, she lives in a wheelchair, unable to speak or walk. Her disease is lifelong, without a cure, and has turned her body into a cage. Her neck and shoulder muscles fail to hold her head up, her back caves in under its own weight, and at times, her arms and legs jerk uncontrollably.

I like working with her, and we work well together. She would do anything to please me. Whenever I pass her wheelchair during the day, I stop to talk, laugh, encourage her, and to push her into moving her muscles. I always make it a game. I cup my hand against the side of her head to support the weight. "Get that head up," I tease.

Rachael tries to grin and lift her head, but her muscles often refuse.

Today I stuck my hands on my hips, thrust my face into hers, and spoke louder, my orders mock serious. "Did you hear me, young lady? Come on, get your head up off that shoulder."

She strained to move her head. I smiled encouragement, but inside I knew how hard she was working. Getting those muscles to obey was difficult.

"Nope! I didn't see that head move at all. You're just playing with me. I know you can do it. Now let's see you. Not bad, not bad, but I know you can do better than that. Come on . . . that's it! That's it! Good girl!"

I work with her on the floor mats as often as I can. I don't like the men on the staff lifting her, because she has to be held under her breasts, and I know she would be embarrassed. One day I lifted her out of the wheelchair and wrapped my arms around her chest from the back to move her to the couch. I didn't realize it, but her shirt had ridden up in the front. It was only when she tried to pull it down that I understood. As palsied as she was, she had still tried to cover herself. She was embarrassed, just as I would be. Although she has Down syndrome, she's high functioning and quite aware of what's going on. Her biggest handicap is physical.

Sometimes my staff forgets that.

I hoisted Rachael out of her wheelchair and flopped down on the couch with her in my arms. Then I wrestled her into a sitting position and propped her up with pillows so she could sit up. I looked at one of the women on the staff. "When was the last time you had her out of this chair?"

There was no answer.

"You have to put yourself in her place. What would you want? Wouldn't you rather sit on the couch than in a wheelchair? Of course, you would. Well, so would she."

When Rachael and I exercise on the mat, I'm always aware of how difficult and how tiring it is for her. The exercises aren't much different from the techniques I use with a six-month-old baby, but they are much harder for Rachael. I lean my whole body against hers, so she feels my strength. I like to think it gives her courage. Trying repeatedly to use a weak arm or leg drains her, so she and I work for only twenty minutes at a time. But even in that short period, when we're finished, she's exhausted.

I know she understands everything I say but is unable to talk to me without her computer, and her spastic hands make even that a problem. I want to be able to talk to her about things that interest her, so I drop in at the public school she attends and pick up tidbits about what's going on in her life. When I learned from one of her teachers that Rachael was being laughed at and ridiculed in her special education class, I transferred her to a school for the profoundly handicapped, something I'd never done before. Now she receives speech and occupational therapy, and she eats her meals with people who never stare or taunt her. She is much happier.

Once Rachael was exercised and back in her chair, I realized I was hungry. I hurried to my office and found my entire family, including my mother, waiting for me to go to dinner. As soon as I walked into the room, Mike threw me a look. "Cooch!" he cautioned.

We were careful when Mom visited, always worried that one of the children like Sandy would throw one of her screaming fits. It upsets some people when that happens.

Mental retardation was largely ignored when my mom was growing up, and Down syndrome rarely mentioned. Not unusual really. Before antibiotics, Down syndrome children seldom lived beyond the age of nine, and most of those young years were spent in state institutions, living in limbo, abandoned, and forgotten. They were called mongolian idiots. With their wide-bridged noses and narrow eyes, like those exotic-looking people from Mongolia, scientists thought these children were a return to a more primitive racial type. People were afraid of them. I was always told it was bad luck to let your gaze linger on a mongoloid.

For some people, even today, watching these children must be like staring at a piece of modern art that is different and dissonant and unattractive until you take the time to learn about it. Of course, many people refuse to take the time.

Just as I reached for my things to go to dinner, Penny walked in carrying Meredith, barely three months old. She is black with a short Afro, a wonderful personality, and a terrible cleft face, so deformed it's as if the corners of her mouth are trying to meet her bottom eyelids. It is so alien a face that it is impossible to take it in all at once. A visitor's mind can only accept the sight in stages: first the eyes, round and brown and unblinking, then the nose, as if there is a segment of a nose on top of a nose, and finally, the split and distorted mouth. She is so deformed that it took three months to find a family to adopt her.

Meredith's mother had been a cocaine addict during her pregnancy, and Meredith was in bad physical shape when she was born. For her to eat, the doctors put a tube in her. For her to breathe, they put in a tracheotomy. Everybody asks me why the doctors bothered. Was she ever going to be happy? How did I know? If she turns out to be retarded, and I still don't have the answer to that, she will never know how ugly she is. If she is normal, won't that be worse? I don't have the answers. We are so used to her that we don't see it anymore, but we know to others she looks like a monster.

As Penny handed the baby to me, my mother shot one quick look at the child and briefly closed her eyes before she turned and walked out of the room. "I'm sorry, I'm sorry," she apologized over her shoulder as she left, but it didn't help. It hurts my feelings when someone won't look at one of my children. I'm not raising monsters—these are my kids.

"Mom, Mom, come back here," I yelled. "I'll hold her this way, turned away from you. Look, all you can see is the back of her head. It's fine."

Mom came back, but she stayed in the doorway, her face troubled. My mother is not the only person who is afraid to look at this child. It isn't an unusual scene around Meredith. Many people don't want to look at her. But my children think she's perfect. We don't see her flaws, so no one else in the room paid much attention.

"Here, look at Carmelo," Jaclyn the peacemaker said to her grandmother. "He's so cute."

"I had almost forgotten him," I said. "Look at that, sound

asleep in his infant seat. This is Carmelo, another one of my cocaine babies."

"He's adorable," Mom said. "He looks perfectly normal."

"He's not. Carmelo's mother had been addicted to crack cocaine for years, and this baby was the first and only live birth in eleven pregnancies."

My mother gasped.

"Every other pregnancy ended in miscarriage or stillbirth. Carmelo was born with a heart defect, Down syndrome, a terrible lung disorder, severe croup, and asthma.

"He was also addicted to cocaine and in withdrawal before he left the birth canal. This little guy weighed only three pounds when he took his first breath. Three pounds, Mother. He might be cute now, but what a mess he was! And he's more nervous and jumpy than any baby I have ever seen."

"How did he get here? And how in the world can you help a baby like that, Camille?" my mother asked. "Sometimes I guess I just don't understand."

"First, I took him because I was told to. He was court ordered here. The judge said, 'Give this baby to Camille Geraldi.' And that was it. Just getting him here helped Carmelo. Second, when I found out he was going to be placed with us, I knew he needed to gain weight before the hospital would release him. So I commuted two hours to the hospital each night after the kids were asleep. That way I could feed him at least one good meal a day. It helped. And we help him now that he's with us. He eats better here than he would have eaten anywhere else, because we work with him."

Mike bent down and laid his hand on Carmelo's forehead. "You're a nightmare to feed, though, aren't you? Sometimes it takes so long to feed him that Bill and Camille have to do it in shifts. But he's cute." My husband the diplomat lifted the baby out of the infant seat and held him toward my mother.

Mom smiled and reached for Carmelo.

Carmelo is named after my grandfather, but with his spiky blond hair and long, skinny body, he certainly doesn't look like my grandfather. I couldn't decide if he resembled a punk rocker or a toothbrush. It didn't matter. Tonight he made my mother smile.

11 Our Trip to Ohio

The Harrison Church Youth Group in Ohio would make my mother smile. They contribute to the foundation not just with their letters and their money, but with their love and support. We were visiting them and having a wonderful time. My mother should have been involved with people like this when she was growing up. She wouldn't be so anxious with Meredith today.

The kids and I sat at a long, low table in the church dining room. In matching blue-and-red shirts, we waited for our meal with folded hands. The only upstart was Matthew, who was beating on the table, his red baseball hat parked backward on his head. With his fringe of dark hair, he was our Italian monk. But no matter how cute he was, he had to mind. I wanted them all on their best behavior.

"Children, remember, our hands go like this." I folded my hands again and bent my head. "Amen. In the name of the Father . . ." I glanced around. No one was paying any attention.

"Excuse me," I said, and waited until I had their attention. Then we finished grace.

As the kids ate breakfast, I walked behind them, making sure they didn't leave a mess. Seth grinned up at me, and I had to smile. One of the girls had stuck his baseball hat on backward like Matthew's. I kissed him on the nose. He was a doll. "What a good boy you are!"

Sitting next to him, Champ caught my eye and pointed to his chest. He wanted to be included. "You too!" I leaned over and planted a kiss on his nose.

After the meal, the young children from the church, dressed in their Sunday clothes, sang a song for us. "If you're happy and you know it, clap your hands." Each line was followed by big claps.

My children, still at the table, smiled at the noise, but no one moved. Were they bored or tired?

"If you're happy and you know it, stomp your feet." The singers stomped their feet.

Now that was more like it! Things were getting better. The Geraldi children stomped on the floor. Those whose feet didn't reach the floor stomped up and kicked the underside of the table.

The singers moved on to the next verse. They stopped stomping. "If you're happy and you know it shout amen. Amen!"

My children lost interest as soon as the stomping stopped, because they didn't know the song. They just watched. At home, if we let them, they would listen to music all day. Singing is probably their favorite pastime. The staff plays all kinds of music, and when they sing, they use big gestures and exaggerated facial expressions that the kids love to imitate. Even the adults with special needs mouth the words to the children's songs or sing right along with the rest of the group. For most of them, singing is easier than speaking.

Other women from the church not involved in the activities sat at long tables on the side of the room. Tan and smiling, delighted to have us there, they talked among themselves and pointed to the different children they recognized from pictures we had sent. They seemed at ease and comfortable with Down syndrome. I was glad for their children's sake.

We put all the children together on the floor, mixing our children and theirs in a circle. They sat cross-legged, their boys in crewcuts and short-sleeved white shirts, their girls in piqué dresses with big sashes and immaculate white anklets. My crew was a lot more casual, but just as neat. When we sang several of our songs for them, they joined in if they knew one, and sang just as loudly and off-key as we did.

My little ones broke the ice for the rest of us. Soon the girls were smiling and cooing at Adelle's and Seth's antics. When Champ elbowed the boy next to him, the boy, startled for a second, quickly recovered his poise and smiled shyly. Then he nudged Champ back. Champ beamed and started telling the kid something. He gestured wildly and bobbed his head up and down in his eagerness. I couldn't figure out what he was saying, but the other boy kept his eyes on Champ and tried to understand.

Matthew, in love with everyone and everything, rested his cheek against a young girl's back as we sang. Her eyes widened in surprise, and she sat up straight, her back stiff. Matthew closed his eyes in bliss, but she didn't move away. If only everyone could have seen the two of them. Here in this room, Matthew was teaching that little girl to look beyond his strange eyes and flat nose. Music was their common denominator, the mutual ground where they could meet and make that first connection, the first awareness that, in some ways, they were alike. I was sure that young girl would remember this moment. Their young age helped, because the older they get, the more difficult it becomes. Champ and Matthew wouldn't be as cute, and others not as understanding.

When the group sing was over and everybody was milling about, Jaclyn sat down on the floor. Her hair was short and tucked behind her ears, not as carefully combed as usual, and she wore as many pierced earrings as Penny. I hadn't realized how much she resembled a hippie until that day. Ever since she got that tattoo on her ankle! Maybe I should say something to her.

It concerned me. I was getting a little alarmed at her appearance when I saw her beckon to Adelle across the room and purse her lips for a kiss. With these kids, Jaclyn never held back in front of other people; she was never embarrassed by their observations or by her own actions. As soon as Adelle saw Jaclyn motion to her, she ran over, planted a juicy kiss halfway between Jaclyn's nose and mouth, then laid her face against her sister's and held the kiss. They stayed together like that for a long moment, arms at their sides, their faces touching, pressed tight against one another.

I wished for my camera. My toddler and my tattooed teenager, her face thinner and more mature, grown up over-night it seemed, showing so much affection in front of strangers. Sisters in every way, bonded and bound together. Sisters in more ways than most sisters. I guess I didn't need to speak to Jaclyn after all.

We spent the long, hot afternoon playing and getting ac-quainted in the backyard of a church member's house. The children were tired and quiet, exhausted from the trip and the heat. I was glad. There was an unfenced swimming pool in the center of the yard. I hadn't forgotten Darlene's ad-venture in a swimming pool, and I have one rule around water. I never let them near a pool or any water unless each child is accompanied by an adult. I never take care of a child myself. My job is to count heads continually and constantly. This trip, we didn't have enough adults to cover the num-ber of children. So even though the weather was hot, there would be no swimming.

I counted heads out of habit. "Where's Matthew?" I hollered. I didn't see him anywhere.

Rosie grabbed my arm and pointed to the porch. "There he is. See?"

Matthew was sitting at the picnic table, his cheek on the tabletop, his eyes at half mast. I breathed a sigh. I should have known better. Rosie, one of my best employees, would never let anything happen to these children, especially Matthew. He was her main man, the first child at the foundation who had smiled at her. On a chain around her neck, she wore a baby charm of his. She never took it off.

Penny, Rosie, and some of the others stayed with me by the pool, their backs to the water. Bill sat quietly by the diving board. New situations like this are hard for all of us. We are more comfortable at home in our everyday routine. Although I act sure of myself, new places and people make me as nervous as anyone else. At home, we are safe and protected, guarded by our rules, anchored to our lives by our hours and our chores. Like the children, we respond to discipline. We are at our best when we have limits. Away from that familiar world, we are different people. How different depends on how secure each of us is within. I walked toward Bill to keep him company.

*T*hree days later, I was back home and busy. Today was Champ's first dancing class, and I wanted to take some photographs. I try to involve the children in some sort of dance or exercise class. Any exercise is good for them, especially one that uses the large muscle groups. Sometimes it's a chore for them, but Champ just happened to get lucky. He was the only boy in his class.

"Curve your arms and make a bubble," the instructor told the children. She had to raise her voice over the classical music in the background.

This room was lovely . . . gray walls with pale-pink trim

. . . polished wood floor . . . little girls in pink leotards and ponytails. I could have stayed there all day.

"Be beautiful ballerinas now. Curve your arms and make your bubbles." The class held their arms overhead in wide, graceful arcs, while my ballet dancer in electric blue tights lay on his stomach on the floor, his chin propped in his hands, daydreaming right in the middle of two dozen five-year-old girls who were trying to ignore him and not trip over him at the same time.

Champ hopped up and took off, and the instructor took off after him. He ran head down, pumping his arms. Then he threw himself on the floor and laughed.

"Champ, all right now, stand up."

Champ never moved.

"Champ, get up please." The instructor started toward him, and he jumped up and scampered back to his place in line. As soon as she turned away, he started clowning around.

"Pssst!" I tried to get his attention.

"Feet together, girls. Knees straight." Champ bent his knees.

"Champ!"

He stuck his thumb in his mouth, chastened for a moment.

That went on for half an hour. He and I were definitely going to have a talk when we got home. As the group danced by me, I pulled my camera out and snapped a quick picture of him. He turned toward the sound of the shutter clicking and waved.

"Bubble arms, remember, bubble arms. Take your bubble to the right, to the left. Lift your bubble over your head and hold it. Hold it. Hold that bubble." As the instructor led the class, a smart aide grabbed Champ's hand and held on to him instead of her bubble. He immediately popped his thumb back in his mouth. I didn't blame him. This bubble talk was boring.

They ended class with a grand promenade around the room. The girls had changed into frilly tutus, and Champ wore a black pirate's hat with a skull and crossbones on the front. I wondered if the instructor was trying to tell me something.

"All right now, lift those arms. Don't crush your tutus. Up on your toes and glide." She started the music.

The class circled the room, arms up, skipping on their toes while Champ ran head down, chin first. I looked away and swallowed a smile. When I glanced back a minute later, Champ was in line with the rest of the dancers, prancing in a circle, on his toes just like the girls. Oh, his hat kept falling in his eyes, but he didn't even stop to take it off.

I couldn't believe it. I beamed, so proud of him for finally behaving. But when the class turned and headed toward my side of the room, I understood. Champ was tiptoeing all over the place like the other kids in his class, not because he loved ballet. And it certainly wasn't because he was going to be another Nureyev. It was simple really. Champ had to go to the bathroom.

12 "*Because the Older They Get . . .*"

John has Down syndrome. He is thirty-three.

His mother, Joan, leaned forward as she talked about him. I had known her ever since I did volunteer work as a teenager and took John for day trips. A small down-to-earth woman, Joan blushed as she talked. She was worried about taking care of her son as she got older. We had been trying to work out a way to ease him gradually into living at the foundation so he wouldn't be so frightened when he finally moved away from his mother.

Joan was perched on the edge of the couch in one of the playrooms. Behind her on a huge bulletin board were hundreds of photographs of everyone who lived at the foundation—kids, adults, and animals. "Of course, it was great for me when you came and took John for a while, because these kids wear you out. When he was with you, I could breathe a little bit." She spoke softly and precisely, her face always composed and pleasant.

I heard her son John shuffling down the hall toward the

. . . .

playroom, following the sound of Joan's voice. When he spotted her, he turned and walked away, content to know where she was.

She lowered her voice and glanced around. "I had been having a lot of problems with John. As he went into puberty, he did some things that weren't acceptable. He was pinching, and doing some other things like that, so he's been to a few schools since the Marian Center. In fact, he's been to many schools. Right now he goes to a workshop for the handicapped during the day. Then he's home with me in the evening."

Brooke and Tiffany hurried into the room to watch a video. They walked to within a foot of the screen before they figured out that the set was not turned on.

"I'm talking, ladies. Out, out!" I cried, and they scooted.

"After our first interview, I decided what I wanted to do about John," Joan said. "You agreed that John could come here and spend the day on weekends. Then, if that works out, and I think it will, he'll start to sleep here one night a week. Eventually, once he's used to it, he'll live here."

I nodded. We had discussed all this before, but I knew she needed to get used to the idea. Hearing the words out loud helped her come to grips with her decision and make it a reality.

"I'd like him to do it gradually. He is so attached to me that I don't think it's good. If I'm not right in sight when he comes in the front door after the workshop, he's yelling, 'Mom! Mom, where are you?' If I leave him with anybody, he's always asking when his Mom is coming home. You know how they get," she whispered.

I did know. It's easy to lose your own life in theirs.

"John was away at a school in Georgia, and they physically mistreated him. So he did everything in his power to come home—pinching people and wetting the bed. Things he had never done before." She held her purse on her lap, fingers gripping the edge, not comfortable talking about her son this way.

"The first time, I brought him here on a Saturday. He was a little bit apprehensive, but he stayed, didn't he? The next week on Friday night, he asks me, 'Am I going to day care tomorrow?' When I asked him if he wanted to go, he got all excited and said, 'Yes!' I was so glad, because I'm getting to the age where . . . oh, John, come on in."

Her grown-up son walked in, flat-footed, head angled to one side, a little like Champ. Shy with dark hair and round brown eyes blinking behind thick glasses, he headed straight for his mother. He sat down near Joan on the couch and stared at the floor. She patted his arm as she talked.

"You don't seem to have any problem at all with the kids here, do you? My heavens, your word is law. They always know what they can get away with, don't they?" She lowered her voice again and glanced at my ankles. "You know, I've known you a long time, and I never noticed before that you wear ankle bracelets. Is that a new style?"

I looked down at my ankle bracelets. "They were the girls' baby necklaces. That's why I wear them. See? One has

. . . .

hearts on it, and one has squares. They're supposed to make your legs look—" I glanced around the room and leaned close to her. "—sexy."

Joan blushed and pushed me away with a laugh.

"And why shouldn't a mother with all these kids look sexy?" I teased.

Alarmed at his mother's laughter, John frowned. "What time we go home?"

She patted his arm again and replied with all the patience in the world, "Just as soon as I'm done talking, we can go, okay? We'll go to the Red Lobster for dinner? You like to eat there, don't you?"

"Sure." He sounded doubtful.

She laughed, and John darted glances at her from out of the corner of his eye. He didn't like to see her occupied with someone else. He muttered under his breath in a fast buzz-saw undertone. "Aunt Katie, I can't wait until she comes down." His diction was rhythmic and almost clear, the way you might sound if you spoke with a face mask on, the skin around your lips stiff and set.

Engrossed in her conversation, Joan merely laid a hand on his knee.

"Okay, kids," he said flatly, not satisfied at all with the amount of attention his mother was paying him. Joan rolled her eyes and tried to finish a sentence. "Sometimes we eat—"

"We go home now?" John asked sly as a fox, looking at her out of the corner of his eye. "I have a—" He thought for

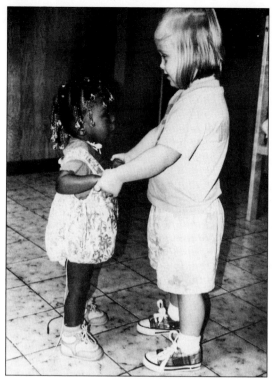

Meredith and Kellie-Ann.

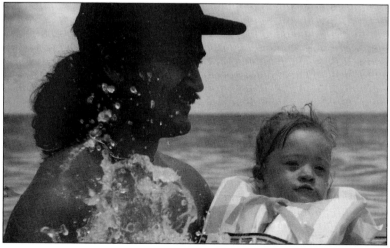

Henry and Adelle.

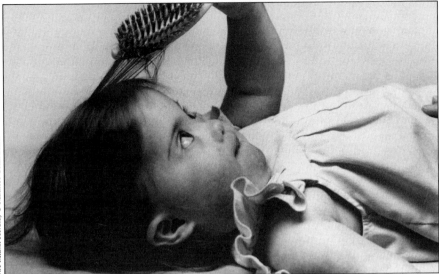

Jo-Layne.

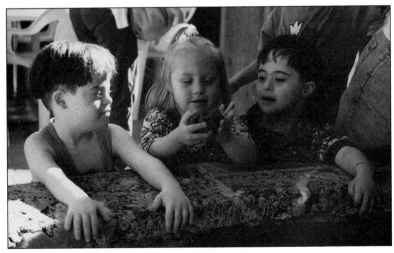

Seth, Kellie-Ann, and Matt at Seaquarium.

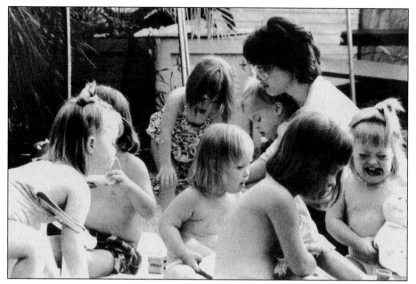

The kids and Wendy lived on the patio for a short time
after the big hurricane.

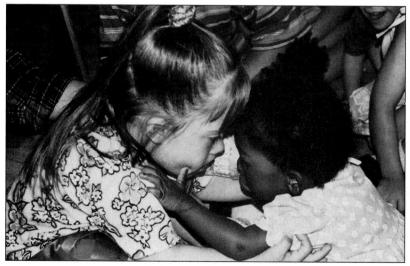

Jo-Layne and Meredith.

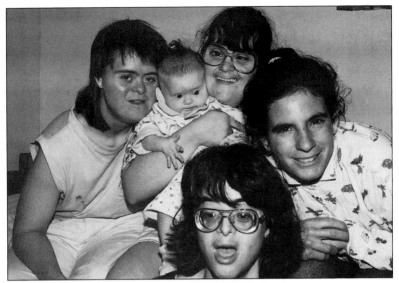

Clockwise, from left: Joanne, Marci, Wendy, and Leeanne.

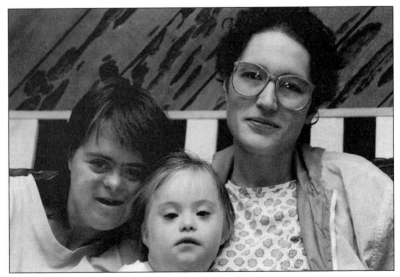

Joanne, Courtney, and Tricia.

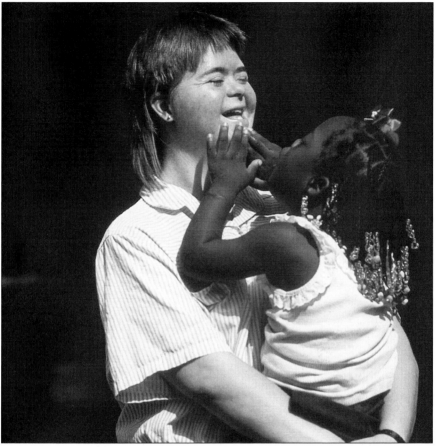

Joanne and Mariah.

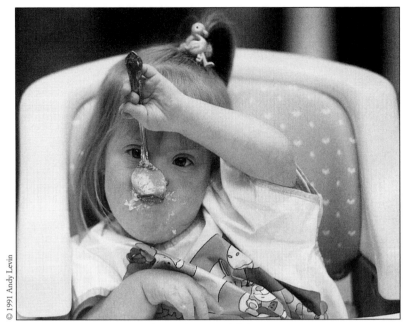

Karley with a mouthful.

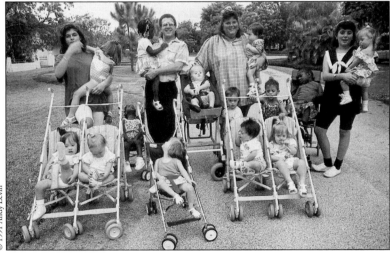

Rene, Mike, Camille, and Jaclyn with some of the kids.

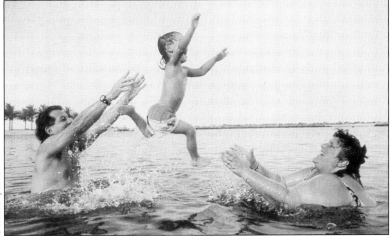

Mike, Champ, and Camille.

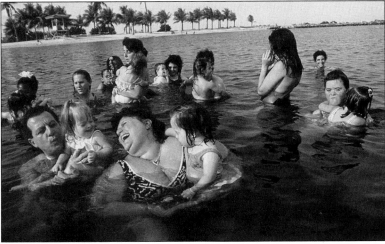

Camille and Mike and their very own water babies.

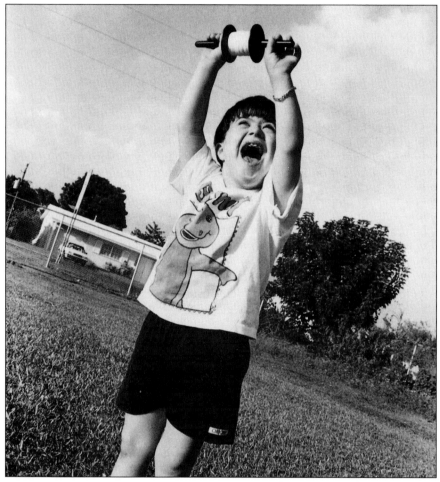

Matthew and his first kite.

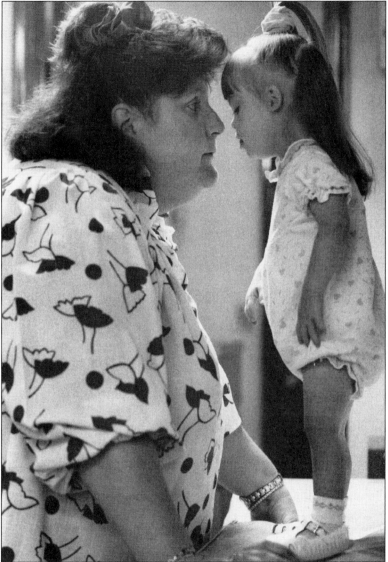

Camille and Brooke.

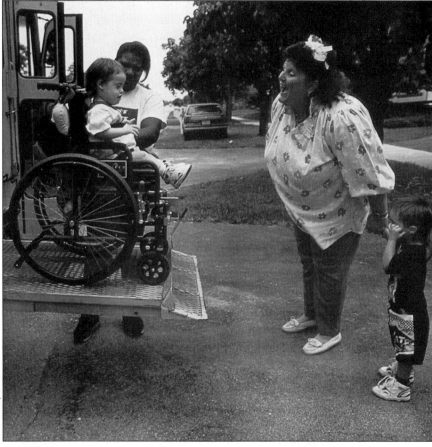

Another exciting school bus ride.

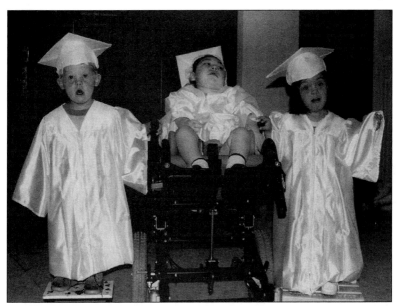

Sonny, Adam, and Angelica at graduation.

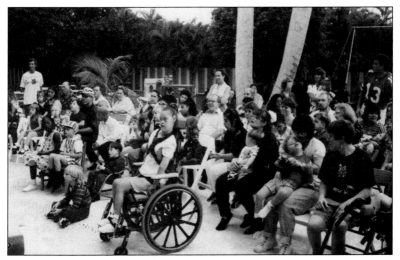

Christmas party, 1995.

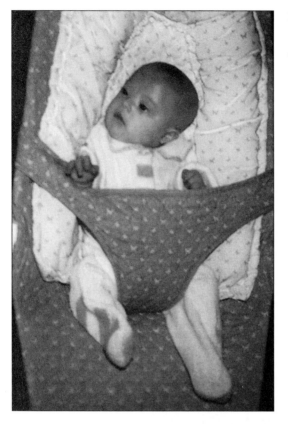

Henry's daughter Joelle.

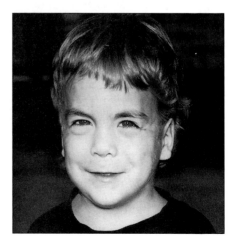

Kyle.

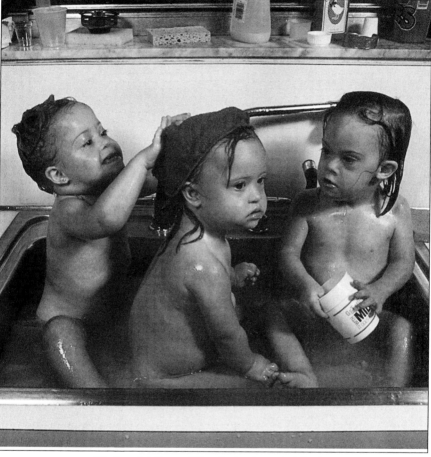

Karley, Adelle, and Brooke having a sink bath.

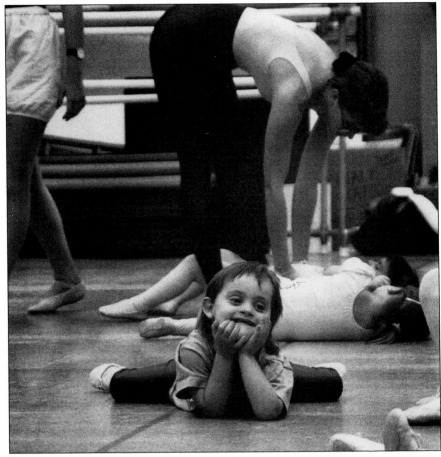

Champ at ballet class.

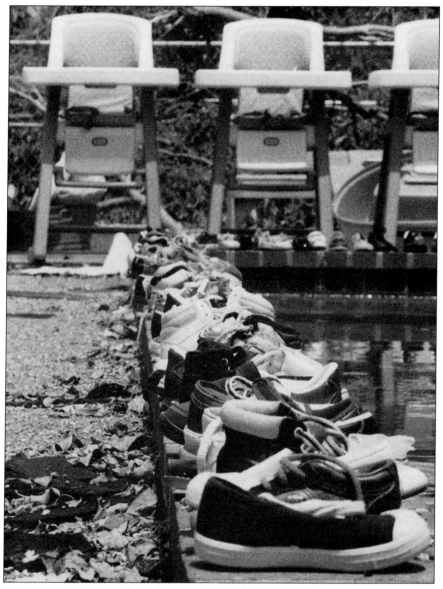

Shoes drying out around the pool after
Hurricane Andrew.

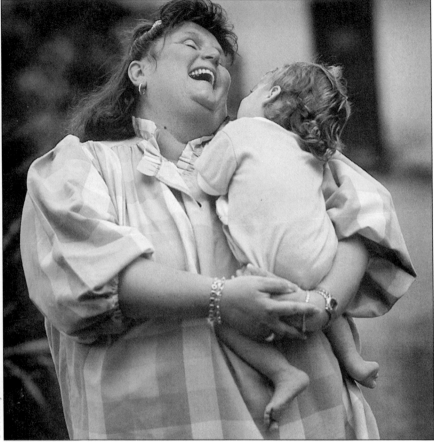

Camille and a little one sharing a private moment.

. . . .

a minute, like a small child trying to dream up an excuse. "—I have a little headache."

It didn't seem to bother Joan. She smiled at his trick and stood up. On his feet in a second, happy and eager again, John waited right next to his mother. Joan was sixty-five and John was thirty-three, and I was sure she was doing the right thing to bring him to us. More important, *she* believed it was the right thing.

As they walked to the door, Teresa's words about her son Kyle floated soundlessly through the air. "I know that if I die tomorrow, I won't have to worry about him."

The Down syndrome adults who live with me now are Wendy, Leanne, and Joanne. Two others who live here, Marci and Tricia, have their own particular neurological deficits. Dark-haired with bright, brown eyes, Marci can be difficult. Her time here with us is the longest she has ever spent in one place. One day when Marci's mother was visiting, she watched her daughter, a bleak expression on her face. "Marci's thirty-two years old, and in all her life, she's never been kissed by anyone but me."

While the special needs adults are part of my family, they are also paid workers at the foundation. There are four of them. Tricia has lived with us for five years. Slim and blond, with none of the physical characteristics present with Down syndrome, Tricia has come a long way since she arrived. She feeds the kids, tends to some of the other routine childcare chores, and proudly handles some of the medications and the feeding tubes. She is the "night supervisor," a title I gave her, but like the others, she is supervised.

I overheard Mike talking to a visitor one day. "If I were to feel sorry for anyone, it would be Tricia. As an infant, she had a seizure disorder that resulted in mental retardation. Her IQ is seventy-eight, so she's higher functioning than the others, yet she's certainly not normal. Tricia lives in between two worlds, the 'normal' world the rest of us live in and the world of the severely retarded. And she knows it. She lives in what she calls the ozone layer."

When Courtney went through a spell of seizures when she was a year old, Tricia wouldn't let anybody else near her. Tricia figured she was the expert on seizures, and she was the one best qualified to take care of Courtney. The two of them bonded better than the strongest glue. They were inseparable.

Joanne, a Down syndrome adult in her twenties, is taller and more evenly proportioned than most Down adults. Quiet, with a sweet face, she has a fine, red rash that spreads across her cheeks like a blush. Her job at the foundation is to help with the young children. Endlessly patient, she always has one of the kids with her.

Sandy, one of my brain-damaged children, often falls into an out-of-control rage. Tall and strong, her hair in perfect cornrows, she turns into another person during a tantrum. Arms crossed over her chest, face contorted and ugly, she arches her back and screams through tightly clenched teeth, silent only when she draws a breath.

One morning after a typical episode, she was lying on her back in Joanne's lap, knees drawn up, ankles crossed. A little girl in a lavender dress with strawberries all over it, she glared at me with real malice when I tried to approach. I stood there quietly and watched.

"Sandy, Sandy," Joanne said, patting Sandy's back over and over again. Her voice droned on, monotonous. As the two of them sat there on the floor, Joanne repeated Sandy's name dozens of times while she stroked her back. The toddler drew sigh after shuddering sigh and finally quieted.

*D*ark-haired, dark-eyed Wendy is the talker in the group. Persistent, often relentless, she pesters everyone with questions and comments. She has also appointed herself our official swimming pool inspector. One day after a storm had filled the pool in our backyard with leaves, Wendy called to Bill. "Pool dirty, Bill."

"Yeah, I know. I know," Bill replied. "Don't get started, Wendy. You only have to tell me once."

"Okay."

An hour later.

"Pool dirty, Bill."

*L*eanne, short, stocky, and thirty-one years old, wears glasses that magnify her eyes and give her a startled expression until she smiles her silly, innocent smile. One of nine children, she was born in the early sixties, a twin, the second set of twins in the family.

. . . .

"Leanne's our ladychild," her older sister Nancy said with an affectionate smile.

After Leanne's birth, the doctors told her father that she probably would not live long. "He took us for a ride in the station wagon and told all of us at the same time that she was dead," her sister said. "We were never to mention her name to our mother again. It would upset her too much. So we never did."

In those years, that wasn't an unusual practice. Over the objections of his wife, Leanne's father secretly placed her in a foster home. When he died many years later, he left his wife seriously ill and speechless from a stroke. As the family sorted through their father's papers, they were shocked to find evidence that Leanne was still alive. They immediately confronted their mother. Unable to speak, their mother spelled out, "Please find her."

With luck from the gods and a little help from the Social Security Administration, they found Leanne living in a group home thirteen miles down a dirt road with a dozen severely retarded children and another Down syndrome adult, Joanne. The two women had been together for seventeen years. Leanne and Joanne were the children's caretakers. The family felt they couldn't separate them, so they found us. Now Leanne and her sister visit and giggle—and share a relationship denied them for thirty years.

When you walk into my house and look at the love Leanne and Joanne and the others have for my other children, I'm sorry, but you can't get that from a normal person. They sit and work with the children all day. They clean and change the gauze around the children's tracheostomies (permanent tracheotomies) so the kids don't develop a rash. They even handle some of the feedings. You should see them—they think they're such big canaries holding up the feeding tubes. Of course, I still can't always understand what they're saying.

It's difficult for many people to understand the adults. The specialized speech training that is available now for Down syndrome children was not around when Leanne and the others were growing up. "Try it another way," I tell Leanne when I can't understand her. Then when she does, often I still don't understand. Usually, we have to ask Penny. We joke and tell her that she's our adult speech specialist. Our ASS.

And although we kid about it among ourselves, the speech of people with Down syndrome is one of the barriers to the so-called normal world. Not only do they not look like everyone else, they don't sound like everyone else, and that frightens people. Many times when I shop in a grocery store with the adults, I notice people turn away from us. As soon as they spot our little group, they head down another aisle. Teenagers are the worst. They say such nasty things.

"Retards!" a group of teenagers yelled one night in the mall. "Just a bunch of retards."

Adults aren't much better. I remember an attorney who told me on the phone that he could help us with a problem.

. . . .

But when we met and he saw the children, he changed his mind. Children like mine bother him, he said. Oh, he thought what we were doing was great, but he couldn't help. I understood, didn't I? If it ever happens to him though, you watch, suddenly we will be the most important people in the world.

You can see that the adults with special needs are especially important to me. This facet of the foundation is close to my heart. Eventually, I want to establish adult training programs in the community that will use similar methods to the ones we use with our adults at the foundation. In these programs, geared to Down syndrome adults and other handicapped people in the community, they will learn to integrate, become more active socially, and gain more independence.

In Dade County where I live and Broward County right across the line, there are *no* services for them. Now the Department of Health and Rehabilitative Services (HRS) is trying to stick them in group homes. They think someone like Leanne is competent enough to live with a small group of handicapped adults like herself. They think these adults can run their own home, without live-in supervision, pay their own bills, and buy their own groceries. I know how Leanne handles money. If she lives in a group home, Leanne will be broke, and probably worse off, because she'll open her door to anyone.

I believe a group home with live-in adult supervision is a sensible answer for adults with Down syndrome, but it's not the only answer. Adults with Down syndrome can live in loving, semi-independent relationships with their birth families. They can live and work in public or private environments similar to ours at the foundation. I know finding these homes is not as simple as it sounds. But it's not an insurmountable problem.

Look at the medical community and the enormous success it has achieved in treating many of the physical problems associated with Down syndrome, particularly heart defects. Look at the government and the wonderful legislation it passed (P.L.94-142, a federal law that guarantees an education to *all* children with handicaps from the age of three to twenty-one).

We as a nation recognize that people with handicaps have their own special needs. What we seem to forget is that they are also citizens with very defined rights and privileges. We fail to understand that they have the right not just to health care or to an education, but the right to live their lives as fully and independently as they can. They have the right to be protected. They have the right to their own personal dignity. They have every single right you and I have.

13 The First Day of School

❧

The minute I bring a new child home, I sign him or her up with HRS. Because the children always have so many medical problems, they qualify for Home Bound, the state-sponsored, home-based school program. If they aren't sick, they go to a school-based program for the handicapped. Under federal law, when they turn three, they go to public school, but they are always in special education classes.

There are three categories of classes: trainable mentally handicapped, educable mentally handicapped, and profoundly mentally handicapped. What category the school system places you in depends on IQ. IQ tests are graded too high. Psychologists dealing with upset parents seem to use a higher score to offer the parent some hope. As a result, the kids get lost in school. They're behind before they ever get started.

Not my bunch! They are always ready.

It was the first day of school, and everyone had been up

since the crack of dawn. The room was full of staff and volunteers, one per child this morning. They waited, each of their charges just about ready. We needed all this help today because the kids took different school buses at different times, one group at 6:45, then another group twenty minutes later.

Angelica, Kellie-Ann, and a few others were still in their high chairs. Karley was even ahead of schedule. She was fed, dressed, hair combed, and ready, well, not exactly ready. Karley wasn't used to getting up quite this early, so as she sat in her high chair, watching the others scurry about, she sucked the thumb on her left hand and leaned her cheek on her right. What was school anyway? Karley closed her eyes. Bed sounded like a better idea.

Not to Champ. Outfitted in Day-Glo shorts, he was just finishing breakfast. All he needed was to have someone comb his hair, and he was out the door.

"You going to school today?" Rosie asked. His eyes were wide with anticipation as he spooned cereal into his mouth and nodded.

"Brooke, are you going to school?" Rosie called. Tricia was through getting Brooke dressed, but Brooke's hair was still wet from her bath. She smiled, baggy-eyed but raring to go. Brooke had a sweet, elfin smile that waited until the last minute, then curled up at the edges. When Tricia stood her up to put the finishing touches on her outfit, the sunsuit straps were too long, and the top of the sunsuit slipped to her waist. Brooke patted her bare chest, trying to figure out what was wrong. She looked at Tricia, waiting for her to notice. Surely she wasn't going to school topless.

Mariah wandered through the kitchen in her nightgown and floppy slippers. "Mariah, school?" Rosie asked as she bent down to give her a hug.

Mariah stuck her nose in Rosie's face belligerently. "No."

I watched the staff get the children ready. The night before, we had packed their backpacks. There were eleven children going to school that morning, so that figured out to be fifty-five diapers, eleven snacks, eleven sets of jumbo crayons, eleven changes of clothing, eleven bibs, Baby Wipes, plastic pants, and underwear! And everything had to be gathered, marked, and packed.

Champ, Karley, and four others were in the first group to leave. This part of the day had to run like clockwork, or we were all in trouble. As I kept an eye on things, I brushed Tiffany's hair. I scooped it up in a ponytail on top of her head, tied a ribbon around it, and stood back to check how she looked. "You're such a pretty girl, Tiffany Geraldi. Do you know how much Mommy loves you?"

A yellow bus drove past the window. "Holy Moses!" I cried. "Look how many buses are going already. That's the second one, and it's not even quarter to seven." I groaned and shook my head. "It's awful to have to go to school this early."

Bill stuck his head around the corner. "Hey, Camille, the school just called. The children have to have mats to nap on by tomorrow." He quickly disappeared.

"Eleven mats by tomorrow?" I asked myself.

A volunteer grabbed Champ and moussed his hair.

When she finished, Champ walked over to Jaclyn with a smile and shyly patted his hair. "Look," he exclaimed with wonder in his voice. His hair stuck up all over his head in trendy spikes.

"A punker!"

"Kyle?" Champ asked as he glanced around. He wanted to show his hair to his brother.

"Kyle's not going to school. He doesn't feel good today," I explained. "He's going to the hospital—"

"Six forty-five!" Eunice yelled. "Let's go."

Jaclyn helped Karley through the back door. Karley was not awake. Then Brooke left with Tricia holding her hand and carrying Brooke's backpack. Then Tiffany and Champ, both hurrying eagerly, went out. Mariah was last, looking not too pleased at whatever was going on. As Renae walked her down the driveway, Mariah tugged at Renae's hand and looked longingly back over her shoulder at the house.

Karley plopped down at the edge of the driveway.

"Stand up!" Jaclyn yelled. "Don't get dirty."

I hurried after the children and tried to remind my daughter about the neighbors. "Jaclyn, people are still sleeping, and there you are screaming."

Champ grabbed Tiffany's book bag and put it in a line with the others. Tiffany's face collapsed.

"Champ, give her that bag!" I pulled my camera out of my pocket and took a picture of their frowning faces.

The other children crowded together, excited at their ad-venture. But not Karley, who sat on the sidewalk again and untied her shoe. She definitely knew something was up, but she was pretending indifference, hoping that would work.

Champ's cool, homeboy shorts, loose and long, the latest style, hung almost to his ankles.

"Where's the bus?" Bill groused, searching up and down the street.

"Oh, it'll be late. It's the first day," I explained. I had been through many first days of school.

Mariah sneezed and wiped her nose on her arm.

"That landed on me too!" I laughed as Eunice wiped Mariah's nose. We used more tissues on her than on any other child.

"Karley's upset," Jaclyn whispered, sounding half-upset herself. "She's scared 'cause she's never been to school before."

"Here's the bus," I announced.

"Stay behind me," I called out to the children who had started yelling and clapping the minute they spotted the bus. I walked to the driveway's edge with a noisy line of kids right on my heels. The bus stopped in front of me, and the door opened.

I smiled at the driver and reached for Mariah to hand her up the bus steps. The driver said something I didn't catch. "What?" I asked. I couldn't hear her above the children's noise.

"I said, I want the children in wheelchairs first," she roared.

"What?" I gasped. "The children in—" The children in wheelchairs weren't due to leave for another fifteen minutes. They weren't ready, and now they were all going in the same bus? How would they fit?

Penny stayed with Champ and the others while the rest of us raced back to the house. I was laughing and trying to run at the same time.

"Where's Darlene?" Jaclyn yelled as she burst through the kitchen door and dove for Darlene's wheelchair. "Somebody go grab Dar! Is she ready? Her bus is here! Get all the wheelchair kids!"

A volunteer grabbed Woody off the floor and whipped him into his wheelchair. Buckles and snaps flew shut. Woody was ready and out the door. Now where was Darlene?

"I've got her," Renae shouted as she scooped Darlene up, grabbed her book bag, and hustled out the door. As Renae ran down the driveway, Darlene wrapped her legs around Renae's waist and hung on for dear life. Her little head bobbed on her neck like one of those plastic dogs in the rear window of a '57 Chevy.

I followed them carrying two book bags I had picked up off the floor. I didn't know who they belonged to. "Who has Seth? Where's Courtney?"

Renae handed Darlene to me at the bus and raced back to the house. "I'll go get Courtney." In seconds, Renae was barreling back toward us, shoving Courtney's wheelchair ahead of her. Thank God, the child was strapped in. I chuckled. She still had milk on her chin.

"Has someone got Seth?" I asked.

"Here he is," Eunice yelled. She ran toward us, pushing Seth in his wheelchair. He jiggled and bounced in his chair, grinning at this new game. Unsettled by the chaos and the change in plans, Champ leaned against my leg and sucked his thumb. The kids who were ready first and waiting at the curb did not understand what was going on. They thought they weren't going to school at all now.

Seth was loaded on first. The bus driver backed Seth's wheelchair onto the wheelchair lift at the rear of the bus, locked the wheels, and flipped a switch inside the door. We yelled and waved good-bye and waited for him to wave back. Seth raised his hands from his lap to wave, but as he felt himself, wheelchair and all, lifted off the ground by something he didn't even see, he froze. He stared into space, his attention riveted on this new sensation for ten or fifteen seconds, his mouth open in amazement.

He finally broke into a huge grin and waved good-bye. Seth was going to school.

Soon the other wheelchairs were loaded on, and the driver was ready for the original group. "How do you want them to sit?" she asked me. "Do they fight?"

"They don't fight with me, but I can't tell you what they'll do on the bus." I held Karley in my arms. She had stiffened as soon as she heard the driver's voice. All this was new to her, and she was afraid. "If they start to fight, and you tell them to stop, they will, because I'm very strict and firm with them."

Eunice handed Brooke up to the driver. As the driver reached for Brooke, the child turned away and clutched Eunice's neck.

"Oh, she doesn't want to go," Eunice crooned and hugged her.

"Let her go, Eunice," I said firmly. "She's just afraid. She'll be okay."

I told the driver what to do. "Sit Brooke with Tiffany if you can. She'll take care of Brooke. Where's Champ? Champ, will you take care of Karley on the bus? See?" I held Karley out to him. "She's crying." Karley patted my chest to make sure I was still there while Champ nodded solemn faced at the bottom of the steps.

"In a little while, you'll be at school. Are you excited, Champ?" Renae asked, empathy all over her face. She remembered what it was like to be little. Champ didn't answer. His day was not turning out quite like he had thought it would. The fear was contagious.

I handed a protesting Karley to the driver. "This is Karley. Sit her with Champ, and he'll take care of her." Karley screwed up her face, her eyes flooding with tears, and she looked back at me as she disappeared into the bus. She would be fine. These children had to get used to the real world, and school was the first place to start. Karley would get over being scared when she realized she was with her brothers and sisters. In this family, nobody is ever alone.

Penny helped Champ up the steps. "Champaretti says put me on the bus, don't you, Champie?" As Penny stepped aside, I snapped a picture of my son and yelled to the driver. "He's wonderful. He'll take care of the other ones."

Renae started up the bus steps with Mariah. "Here's . . ."

"This one's still crying," the driver yelled from inside the bus. I pushed Renae aside and hauled myself up the steps. I just stood there in front of the children and let them see me. "Karley? Are you all right? You'll be fine. Tiffany, you take care of her, you hear me?" Tiffany patted her sister's leg and stuck her face in Karley's with a grin.

"Champ, you watch your sisters, all right?"

He nodded, his eyes saucers, still overwhelmed. He was fine.

I climbed down, handed Mariah into the bus, and heaved a sigh. "I'll see you later," I yelled.

"Bye!" Rosie yelled. "See you later."

Everyone yelled and waved, smiling wide smiles of encouragement as the bus pulled away.

"Bye, Seth."

"Good-bye, Champ. Bye, Tiffany."

"See you later, guys."

"See you soon, Karley," Renae cried.

"Bye, bye, bye," I yelled.

Jaclyn tapped my arm. "Mom, the neighbors are trying to sleep."

14 *Discipline and Love*

❧

Our Miami neighborhood looked deserted in the early afternoon sun, and a hot breeze barely stirred the dense shrubbery around the house. The only sounds were the muted rumble of an outbound jet and, out of sight in a back-yard, the slow, steady tick of a sprinkler on a new lawn. Inside our house, it was dark and cool, the house's interior offering a quiet reprieve from the heat. The silence, especially at nap time, astonished visitors.

My sister Jo-Ann and I sat in my office, going over some papers. As we worked, I picked up six-month-old Adam and laid him in my lap. "I think you're doing a little better," I said as I studied his face. I was tracing circles on his back when suddenly a whirlwind burst through the door. The younger children, up from their naps, rushed into the room.

Tiffany made a beeline for me and held out her arm. "Boo-boo, I got a boo-boo," she said dramatically.

"Oh, you're right. Look at that," I commiserated, and she beamed.

Champ tore into the room, marched up to me, and jammed his hands on his hips. He had a video tucked under his arm. "Turtle?" he demanded. I shook my head, and he turned to Jo-Ann, his head tilted to one side. He walked up to her and stood there for a second, a challenging look on his face. Then he leaned in with a laugh and gave her a quick kiss.

"Turtle?" he asked her, no less hopeful this time.

"He wants you to put his Ninja Turtle video on. He asks for that video all the time. Champ, go ask Bill." I pointed to the door.

Before he left, he dashed over to Jo-Layne, who had just stumbled in. When he started to rough-kiss her, she shook her head. Her whisper fine hair whipped around her face. No, thank you. Jo-Layne remembered his head-butting kisses. She had old eyes like Champ's, but the two children weren't alike. He was blustery; she was quiet. He was brazen; she was shy. She leaned against my arm and patted the baby's head. Her eyes stared at something just over my shoulder as if she were remembering. This tough John Wayne kid probably did know things the other children hadn't learned yet.

Champ raced across the room, headed for Bill. "Turtle?" he yelled as he passed the rest of the kids, hurrying through the door.

Karley and Adelle leaned across my knees and faced each other nose to nose as I talked. Dressed alike in peach and blue, they patted and poked each other's faces as they smiled and jabbered together. They would have been content to stay there all day stretched across my lap, propped on their elbows. But after a few minutes, I called Penny to take them. I had things to do.

Even though my family teases me about my attention to detail, I know that my knack for organization keeps everything running smoothly. As I walked through the dining room, I checked the children's charts tacked on the wall. They listed over twenty different educational, social, and physical goals. Kept on file for each child, these charts, called Individual Education Programs, are written and evaluated every other month in our staff meetings. The charts include the work we do here at the foundation. We teach them what all parents teach their children, everything from appropriate social behaviors to the sound a cow makes. But we place special emphasis on speech, cognitive faculties, and large and small motor skills. The charts also include the time spent with speech and physical therapists, and the time in Home Bound, an at-home school taught by a state-funded teacher. At the end of two months, our IEPs are reevaluated, progress reports are written, and new ones are drawn up according to each child's needs.

Champ's chart lists, among other things, speech tapes, swimming lessons, and puzzle play. Darlene has developed much more slowly even though she is a year older. Among her goals are bubble blowing, brushing hair without crying, and stopping herself from hitting herself. Jo-Layne is working on waiting her turn more patiently.

On my right is the children's playroom/dining room. A fifteen-foot closet filled with clothes runs the width of the room. On the floor of the closet dozens of pairs of shoes are lined up perfectly. I have a separate closet for Sunday and holiday clothes.

A high shelf runs around the perimeter of the room, filled with identical white plastic baskets, a child's name on each. In the afternoon, we place their pajamas in the baskets, and at night we put in their clothes for the next day. That way nothing is ever lost or out of place.

I want the children to learn to be neat and responsible. I require a great deal from them. "I expect . . ." is a phrase I use all the time. I expect them to put their things away, to pay attention, to brush their teeth, and to take a bath. I expect it because society expects it. If they can't conform to these basic requirements, how can they get along in a society that is already so biased against them?

Even the adults who came to live with us had to learn the rules. They were not ready for society. Some of them had never been shown the first thing about cleaning or taking care of themselves. Their personal hygiene left a lot to be desired. I shut myself up in the bathroom with each one of them and demonstrated exactly what to do. I showed them how to use a toothbrush, a washcloth, and deodorant.

The little ones had had these lessons drilled into them since they were babies, and they knew what was expected of them. But after their behavior the previous week, perhaps society wasn't ready for them after all.

The kids had climbed off the school bus and were trooping noisily through the house, headed straight for the potty room. They know there are no snacks until that chore is out of the way. So every day they drop their backpacks in a pile and line up for the bathroom. Today, very tired, they whined and argued.

"Mine! That's mine!" Champ yelled, pointing to someone else's backpack. "Mine!"

"Champie, get in line," I said. "That's not yours. Yours is blue. This one's purple."

"Mine!" he insisted, hands on his hips, his chin stuck out belligerently.

I bent down, touched his nose, and asked softly, "Do you want time-out?"

A time-out is three or four minutes of silent time spent isolated from the group. The children hate it. They can't talk or look at any of their brothers or sisters. It isn't a harsh punishment, but it works. It is devastating to these kids. When someone scolds a Down syndrome child, the look on the child's face is so forlorn, the scolding hardly seems worth it.

I'm the first to admit I'm strict, but no member of the staff is ever allowed to hit the children. I taught them to use time-out or a two-fingered tap on the back of a hand when they are really serious. One day I found Christopher tapping the back of his hand. *He* knew when he had done something wrong, even if no one else did.

Uh-oh, I could hear Jaclyn in the next room reprimanding someone.

"Time-out," Jaclyn cried to Adelle after the child had repeatedly ignored her. Adelle dropped to her knees, leaned her forehead against the big TV screen, and shared her time-out space with Vanna White on *Wheel of Fortune.*

Some of them have to be told twice, but as soon as the order *time-out* sinks in, they are at a wall or a door or, as in Adelle's case, forehead to forehead with Vanna. I have even found their dolls sitting on the floor, facing the wall, in time-out.

With a family this size, there have to be some bottom-line rules. Mine are simple: discipline, love, and respect. The children are brought up with physical affection, discipline, and days full of stimulation.

"Well, Champ?" I asked, getting back to my own discipline problem right in front of me. "You haven't answered my question. Do you want time-out?"

Champ shook his head, his chin down, glancing around from underneath his eyelashes to see if anyone was watching. Karley was already in time-out at the sliding glass door a foot away. She hadn't even made it all the way into the potty room before she got in trouble. Sitting on the floor cross-legged, she held on to her feet and stared dejectedly at her ankles.

Her sister Tiffany wasn't that lucky. She was in the kitchen, sulking in her time-out. From her chosen spot under the counter, she darted little glances at what was going on and sniffled.

Not all discipline problems were so easy to handle.

*O*n another afternoon when the kids had just gotten home from school, I heard Penny scolding them. Now

. . . .

what? I asked myself as I followed the sound of her voice. They were all in the kitchen.

"What are you yelling about? I can hear you all the way in my office."

"Look at them," Penny said as she pointed to the sad-looking group in front of her. It was Brooke, Jo-Layne, Courtney, Champ, and Karley. "Do you notice anything?"

"Notice anything?" I asked. "No, I . . .what? Wait a minute. What's going on here?" They still wore their school clothes, schoolbags in their arms, but they didn't have any shoes on.

Penny stood there with her arms folded. "The bus driver told me they threw their shoes out of the bus window."

I couldn't believe it. Their shoes cost a fortune. I planted my hands on my hips and spoke firmly. "Threw them where? Do you know what this means?"

Champ shook his head and sucked his thumb so hard it turned white. Both Karley and Brooke had tears in their eyes, and Jo-Layne was close. If I was going to carry this off, I couldn't look at them, or I would laugh.

"Come with me," I ordered, my voice gruff. They looked at each other and followed me reluctantly to my office. "Here, line up in the hall, one by one. Right outside my door."

Karley tried to pull away, but that didn't work. I pushed and pulled the five of them until they were lined up, standing behind each other just outside the door to my office. Champ's eyes filled his face. They had no idea what was coming.

I went into my office and cried, "Penny, bring me that thing."

Karley frowned and Courtney just stood there with her mouth open. She didn't understand what was happening at all.

"What?" Penny yelled back dramatically. I could just imagine her grin.

"You remember!" I replied. I had to turn away so the kids wouldn't see me smile. But I knew the children heard Penny rummaging around in a kitchen drawer.

After a few seconds, my intercom buzzed.

"Camille, what are you talking about?" Penny asked. "What do you want me to bring?"

"How should I know?" I whispered. "I'm just trying to get their attention. I don't want to scare them to death." I hung up the phone. We weren't very good at this, I decided. All we had mastered were time-out and the two-fingered tap.

I heard Penny hurrying down the hall past the children. She walked into my office and partially closed the door. Shrugging her shoulders, she rolled her eyes and announced, "Here it is."

I looked around. She didn't have anything with her. I held my hands out, palms up. "Here what is?" I whispered. I didn't want the kids out in the hall to hear.

"Here's what you told me to get," she said in a low voice.

I was confused. "I didn't tell you to get anything."

"I know," she replied softly. "That's what I brought."

"That's what you . . . oh, I get it." I grinned. "We just pretend there's a thing? What kind of thing?"

"Camille, I have no idea. Don't start that again." Her face reddened as she tried not to laugh.

"Okay, Penny, call the first one in." I stood in front of my desk and held one finger to my mouth. "Don't you dare laugh," I whispered.

She nodded and opened the door. Standing in the doorway, her face stern, she called for the first culprit. "Champ!"

Champ dragged his heels as he walked into my office. When Penny closed the door behind him and left the other children waiting on the other side, I could hear one of them sniffling. Champ, his thumb still in his mouth, looked everywhere but at me. "Young man, what possessed you to throw your shoes off the bus?"

He shook his head.

"Are you ever going to throw your shoes off the bus again?"

He shook his head harder.

"Never, never do that again! Do you understand me?"

"Yes," he said.

I pretended to think about his situation for a minute. "Okay, then, if you promise me you will never do it again, you can go. Don't stop and talk to the other children. Just go right into the kitchen for your juice, then head over to Rick. He's going to help you color today. But remember what I said."

He nodded and waited for Penny to open the door. When he walked out, she turned her head away from the children and grinned at me.

"Next," I yelled. "Next!"

No one moved.

"Who's next, Penny?"

Penny crooked her finger. "Brooke! Front and center."

We repeated our performance four times. At the end of ten minutes, we were tired, but the kids knew I meant business.

A few minutes later, I followed the children over to the other house to check the menus for the following month. Rick, our fix-it man, was watching the toddlers, a chore he didn't usually handle. As I walked into the room, he was placing sheets of drawing paper in front of them. Heads over their coloring, they giggled and talked to their crayons as much as they did to one another.

"Matt, watch it!" Rick yelled. Matt was leaning too far over the side of his chair. Rick steadied him with one hand and reached across to hand Jo-Layne a piece of paper with the other. His face was beet red.

"Draw me a picture. No, don't eat it!" he said, an incredulous look on his face. "You don't eat them, they're not food."

Jo-Layne watched him like a hawk as he stood up and reached for the box of crayons. She wasn't sure she was going to get another one.

"Here . . . this is green. Draw some grass." He shoved his hat to the back of his head and sighed with exasperation as he sat back down.

Renae interrupted with a tap on the door. "Is it all right if Billy comes outside to feed the animals?" Billy was there for daycare.

"Me?" Champ asked. His face brightened.

"Sure, Renae," Rick nodded. "No, Champ, you wait. You'll go outside later. Who wants another color?" He circled the table, retrieving the old crayons before handing out new ones. "Here's red to go with the green you had, Jo-Layne." The crayon was orange.

Champ watched longingly as Renae left the room.

"Matt, what's the matter?"

The little boy stared straight ahead, pouting.

"You don't like gold?"

Matt shook his head.

"Gold's good." The crayon was brown.

"What'd I hear about you kids and your shoes today, huh?" Nobody said a word. They didn't even look up.

"Threw 'em off the bus?" Rick chuckled. "I did that once. My dad told me later no point in throwing one shoe away. Might as well throw them both out."

"Rick!" I caught his eye and shook my head.

"Well, anyway," he said, hesitating. "Look at these crayons, would you? Now they got skin tones and everything. Hey, Matt, not on the table. You want Mommy to come over here and see that? No? 'No' is right. Okay then. What's wrong, Champ? You don't like yours! Here's a good color," he promised. But the crayon he held up was black.

"Go outside," Champ said softly to himself, sticking his lower lip out.

Next to Rick, Jo-Layne rested her forehead on her arms and dozed off. "Hey, wake up," Rick cried, shaking her arm. She opened her eyes, blinked at him blankly, and closed them again.

"You don't want to draw no more? No problem. Champ,

how about you? Where's your crayon? Don't draw on the table please. Adelle, yellow? Hey, where's your paper? What are you going to color on?" Adelle, her ponytail askew, red crayon on her shirt, pointed to the floor, mystified. "Well, pick it up," he said.

In a better mood now, Champ sang his favorite song. "Happy birthday to you . . ."

Before long, it was dinnertime, and Rick gathered everything up. Jo-Layne's crayon was nowhere to be found. "Don't tell me you ate it," he said. A look crossed her face as if she was wondering the same thing.

"That's it, coloring's over." He had to raise his voice to be heard over the children who were singing along with Champ.

A group of teenage volunteers appeared to pick the children up.

"Go with them, go on now. And you keep your shoes tied, you hear me?" He threw his head back and laughed, ignoring my look.

The next day, I met the school bus myself. As the driver pulled up in front of the driveway, I could see her waving her arm around and saying something. She was already halfway through her sentence when she threw the bus door open.

" . . . not my fault. I can't be looking everywhere at once."

"What?" I asked, alarmed, already halfway up the bus steps. "What's wrong?"

"These damn kids threw their shoes off the bus again!!"

I nodded and held one finger to my lips to silence the children as they trooped slowly off the bus. Karley's socks were filthy, and Jo-Layne only had one on. Champ still had one shoe, and so did Courtney, but the rest of them wore no shoes at all.

Brooke looked up at me and opened her mouth to say something. "Not a word, young lady. Not one word." I shooed them up the driveway to the house, walking behind them and waving my hands as if I were shooing chickens. They banded together in a knot at the door and waited for me to open it.

I watched their faces as I motioned them inside. I knew they had to go to the bathroom; I knew they were starved and thirsty. But they moped along as if they were on the way to the guillotine. I shut the door firmly behind us.

"Penny!"

I was upset that afternoon, but I laughed when I thought about it later. We broke the Geraldi record that day—ten children in time-out at once. The kids had an excuse, though. It was Friday, and we were leaving in a little while for our cabin in North Carolina.

We love spending time there. We can let our hair down and be ourselves. Mike and I hike and swim with the kids. We cook and garage-sale and hunt for antiques. That year we were going to the Sorghum Festival. The cabin is always a relaxing, down-home escape.

We arrived late the following night, too late to unpack. Everyone just unloaded the bus and the van and dropped things anywhere. The room was ringed with boxes and coolers and piles of clothing. Liter bottles of water and soda and juice. A breathing machine. Bags of food. A box of medicine. Sheets and sleeping bags and pillows stuffed everywhere. I was going crazy with the mess.

I stood in the middle of the kitchen, in shorts and a T-shirt, my hair pulled back in a ponytail, half-hidden under a baseball hat. Was I tired! What a long drive from Miami.

"What is Jo-Layne eating?" Renae cried. "Mom, look at her! What's that in her mouth?"

"Banana, Bill just gave all of them some banana. Why?" I bent down and opened Jo-Layne's mouth. "Oh my God, she's eating the peel. Didn't any of you see that?" I picked her up and set her on the kitchen counter. "Open your mouth. No, don't swallow, you little monkey." I started to laugh. "Do you believe this child? Now, open your mouth." I threw the peel away and wiped off her face. "Now where's the rest of the peel?" Renae spotted it on top of the breathing machine.

As I walked through the living room, I saw Bill on the couch, giving Carmelo his bottle. It was hard to believe he had never fed a baby before joining us at the foundation.

"Come on now," he said softly. "We're not getting anywhere at all."

"Which nipple are you using?" I asked.

"The Nuk," he replied, without looking up, his eyes on the baby's face.

For my new babies, Nuk nipples are the best, especially for a Down syndrome infant. We buy them at Eckerd's Drugs

. . . .

and Toys R Us stores. Feeding techniques are extremely important too. When I give a bottle, I hold my little finger under the baby's chin and push gently. It forces the nipple closer to the roof of the baby's mouth and makes it easier to suck. Manipulating and exercising the muscles around the cheeks, above the lip, and under the chin helps too.

Bill sat the baby up and patted his back for a burp. "That's better, isn't it?"

"Are you burping after every ounce?" I asked.

He nodded. "Hear that, little fella? You'd better keep this meal down, or you're in big trouble around here." His voice was gentle.

Later, when the cabin had cooled off, everyone lay on the floor in the living room and watched TV. Or at least, some of them tried. It was hard with five kids piled on Penny's back singing, "The people on the bus go up and down, up and down, up and down . . ."

With each up and down, Penny bucked higher and higher until the kids were squealing so hard they couldn't sing.

"Come on," Jaclyn cried. "The people on the bus go up and down."

Jo-Layne, first in line right on Penny's neck, grabbed Penny's head and held on while Penny bucked. When Champ and Tiffany heard the screams and the laughter, they flew into the room. As they climbed behind Jo-Layne, she slapped them away and hugged Penny's head tighter.

"Solly the Camel has five humps. So ride, Solly, ride. Boom, boom, boom . . ."

. . . .

With each boom, Penny bounced. Adelle clutched Matthew ahead of her and laughed so hard that both of them fell off. I howled. In seconds, they hopped back on. The kids slid and bounced and laughed until Penny collapsed, her face scarlet.

She glanced at me, deadpan. "Camille, these kids have got to go. They're killing me." But Penny didn't fool anybody.

I was still smiling when I put the children to bed. I laid a hand on Adelle's forehead. "Good girl, no fever tonight. That cold's all gone. Now give Mommy a kiss." Adelle's eyes closed before my kiss landed on her cheek.

Jo-Layne had crawled into bed by herself, and I went over to tuck her in. "Are you asleep already?" I leaned over her bed, pulled the rubber band out of her ponytail, and nuzzled her neck. She smelled like toothpaste and banana.

Jaclyn settled Champ down, then turned to me and held out a fist. "I shouldn't laugh. It's not funny. Look what Jo-Layne was just eating."

"If that child was eating banana peel again . . ."

"Nope, this tastes better than that." She opened her hand. Jo-Layne had been eating Legos.

15 The Astronomical Figures

❧

*E*veryone always asks what our expenses are. How much money does it take to run this foundation? Household figures, usually too dull to repeat, become fascinating in a family this large. Our family expenditures in one month include

$1,800 electricity

$2,500 food

$1,200 diapers

$800 clothing

$8,600 medical

Not to mention other personal expenses plus foundation expenses: gas, phones, mortgages, insurance, staff salaries, and, oh, don't forget car insurance. The car pool includes two vans, one bus, a motor home, and five cars. Each month it costs $22,000 to run the family and foundation.

. . . .

And that doesn't include the price of an adoption. The expenses for one adoption procedure run between $6,000 and $10,000.

And food? In a week, this family consumes

18 gallons of milk

28 loaves of bread

10 boxes of cereal

50 jars of baby food

I order my meat and some other frozen foods from a Florida-based company I have used for many years. A typical order includes

12 packages broccoli

36 packages ground beef patties

16 packages ravioli

11 packages chicken nuggets, 48 in a package

20 packages meat balls

35 packages hot dogs

12 packages corn on the cob

I reserve Wednesday nights for pizza. Each week, I order twelve.

The babies aren't so lucky. I seldom feed them solid food the first year. Born with poor digestive systems, the only thing

I find that they tolerate well is liquid Similac at room temperature. It gives their systems time to mature. I feed them whatever amount they will take, but I always feed one ounce and burp. I've found this eliminates the typical stomach problems common to Down syndrome children.

But no matter what their age, food is important to this family. A year ago, when a storm knocked out our power and water for several days, I spent half my time fixing the food.

We roughed it in the backyard, lost without air-conditioning or water. The children wore only diapers or shorts, and I could spot their surgery scars twenty feet away. It was a good thing everyone was well, because we just lined the high chairs up, plopped the kids in, and handed out their meals. If we let them feed themselves as usual, there wouldn't have been enough water to clean them up, so I walked back and forth and fed them from one big bowl.

When they saw me coming, the kids opened their mouths like baby birds. Smiling and laughing as the food headed their way, they had no idea what was going on. I brushed a strand of hair out of Tiffany's eyes and slipped a spoonful of yogurt into her waiting mouth.

"M-m-m," she said, and opened her mouth for more, but I had already moved on to Jo-Layne. Tiffany would have to wait for me to catch her on the return trip. What do truckers say? "Catch you on the flip-flop, Tiffany."

Matthew waited openmouthed next to her, his chest bright red from spilled juice.

"Drink nicely, Matthew," I said. "You don't know when you'll get a bath."

. . . .

With the power out everywhere, people brought food from their freezers, wonderful things like steak and lobster that this crew of mine have seldom eaten. Others brought pans of barbecued ribs, baked ziti, macaroni and cheese, fruit, vegetables, and bread. When I set it out on the table, my adults thought they had died and gone to heaven. "Eat!" I cried, and they did.

I leaned over the table and shook my finger, pretending to scold them. "You're eating the best meals of your lives, do you know that?"

They bobbed their heads and giggled.

"You would sit there and eat for hours if I let you, wouldn't you?" Then I laughed. "I ought to send you a bill."

All of them nodded, laughing with their mouths full.

*I*n the old days, Mike paid all the bills. But that was before we had so many children. Today it's different. Of course, he still contributes, but we also have donations and other sources of income. One of my favorite donations is for $2.50. It comes each month from a woman in Arizona State Prison. It's her monthly salary.

We receive monthly checks to provide for Derrick and Jahida's care, and I apply for grant money to the government, private businesses, and other institutions. Grant proposals are long and involved, and not much fun to do, so I hire grant writers. But grant money isn't constant. Grant funding is not money that I can depend on regularly.

Before Leanne and Joanne came here, they lived in a home

where the caretakers were paid $1,500 a month plus an additional $430 from Social Security for each adult: $1,900 a month! We get nothing. We receive only $430 a month from Social Security, and that does not even pay for all their medicines. It certainly isn't enough to house, feed, and clothe an adult or a child.

Even though I seldom talk about it, money always worries me. I'm always trying to figure out what I would do if the donations and grants stopped. I wish the state did more, but you can't argue with them. All you can do is tolerate the situation. It's ironic. I can't demand anything from the state, yet they make huge demands on me. They wanted overhead sprinklers and fire alarms. I put in overhead sprinklers and fire alarms. Then they wanted special hurricane shutters, or we'd have to go to a shelter during a storm. I had the shutters installed. Then they wanted me to buy a generator. I bought a generator! How can you argue?

*R*enae and Jaclyn were busy unpacking groceries in the pink house while I started dinner. Mike always said watching me put groceries away was mind numbing. Cucumbers went in the refrigerator bin, one by one, lengthwise. I stored cans with every label facing front. When I found a shelf out of order, I pulled all the items out and restacked them.

The girls finished up while I checked supplies on the changing tables down the hall. I don't want to sound like a commercial, but I am particular about which products I use on the children. I have to be. The smallest rash can grow into a monumental medical problem. I have found name-brand diapers and pull-ups (a cross between a diaper and training pants) such as Huggies and Pampers work best. A good quality powder such as Mycostatin, A and D Ointment, and Balmex (made by Block Drug) also work well for us. We couldn't survive without Baby Wipes. If a rash does appear, I switch to tissues and warm water. Nothing else.

As I mentioned earlier, the babies drink liquid Similac only. All the children are given vitamins on a daily basis. Depending on their age, we use Poly-Vi-Flor, Poly-Vi-Sol, Tri-Vi-Flor, and Tri-Vi-Sol.

I wash the infants' clothing myself in Ivory Snow and use Shout on all clothing stains. All the children have baths and shampoos every single day, more often if they need them, and I brush their teeth every chance I get. Too often, Mike says. I probably go through a tube of toothpaste a day. Fingernails and toenails I keep clipped short.

I shop at sales for their clothes and at a secondhand store near our cabin where most of the clothes were outgrown before they were worn. Yet I buy them for only two or three dollars each. I bet I have three hundred outfits to sort through before school starts.

You can see that taking care of these children requires all my time. I wish I had more time to give them. Around my neck I wear a heart with an inscription that says it all: *Twenty-four hours is never enough.*

16 *Dinnertime*

❧

It was almost five thirty, and most of the kids were already seated at the three dining room tables, waiting. The babies were in bed, and the profoundly retarded children had already been fed. I love this part of the house. The room turns gold in the late afternoon as the sun slants through the patio doors and across the wood-paneled walls. That evening, some of the children had their hands pressed together to say grace, and, for an instant, the dining room looked like a church.

Dinner was barbecued chicken, rice, and mixed vegetables, and everyone was hungry. What else was new? Two hours ago, I had assembled the meal: forty-eight pieces of chicken in two pans so big and so heavy that Henry had to lift them into the oven. Before I baked the chicken, I poured barbecue sauce all over the top and filled the gaps with cup after cup of rice. Then I added water until it came to the top of the pan.

As I dragged a ten-quart pot across the surface of the

stove, the phone rang. I listened for a minute, hung up, and made a quick call. When I was finished, I turned to the staff. "There are head lice at the kids' school. I just called Mike's office for the stuff to get rid of them." Amid moans and groans, I laughed. "I wonder why I'm the only one immune to them."

"I know," Henry yelled. "It's all that stuff you put in your hair."

I chuckled at his joke as I dumped the vegetables into the pot. "Quit teasing me about my hair spray." Earlier that week, Adelle had made a face and pulled her hand away when she touched my hair.

"You're immune to everything, Mom," Renae cried. "You never catch anything."

Leanne ignored the teasing and watched her feet as she carried the adults' water glasses to the table, her face serious and determined. It took her many trips to finish the job, but not a drop spilled.

Mike stood behind me at the stove as I cooked, catching me up on his day at the office, while Renae scurried back and forth, fetching and carrying. Hungry eyes followed every plate she brought to the table.

When Mariah got a little too eager and scrambled out of her seat for the kitchen, Jaclyn stepped in. "Remember what Mommy says. If you're not here for dinner, you don't eat," she announced, quoting me. Everyone knew I allowed no eating between meals—at least not from my kitchen.

"Kitchen open!" Jaclyn cried and clapped her hands once. "Kitchen closed!"

No one ate, no one even touched their food until Mike sat down.

"Good manners, Jo-Layne," Bill said when he spotted her waiting patiently.

Rosie coached Matthew when he pointed to a drawing of a car. "Car, say car, Matthew. Come on, say car."

"Car," twenty-eight-year-old Joanne answered softly from the other table. Rosie turned around, surprised. Of all the Down syndrome adults, Joanne was the quietest.

I turned the heat down under the vegetables and picked up Tiffany who was racing by me for the table. "It took you ten minutes to come say hello to Mommy?"

She held her hand over my mouth. "Stop, Mommy."

Two of the kids were singing together, murdering "The Inky Dinky Spider."

The room quieted down. Tonight it was Marci's turn to say grace. Although not Down syndrome, Marci was one of the adults with special neurological needs. Her grace tonight was brief. She was probably exhausted. Earlier, she had spent the afternoon with two of the kids, Derrick and Jahida. Profoundly retarded, they laid curled at her feet on floor mats, their backs curved into fetal positions, unaware of what was going on around them. Marci didn't mind. She was busy teaching them Yiddish.

Before grace, they all blessed themselves. "In the name of the Father . . ." The Church never taught the sign of the cross with more poignancy. I smiled as the tip of a nose, an eyebrow, a forearm, even a knee became a touch point.

Jo-Layne sat in the catbird's seat next to me at the foot of the table. She had a reputation for eating anything, and even though everyone's chicken was cut off the bone, I kept an eye on her while she ate. Jo-Layne was the Geraldi version of a garbage disposal. That wasn't as silly as it sounded. The teacher gave her a plum at school one day. Jo-Layne ate the whole thing, and later, I found the plum pit in her colostomy bag.

Adelle sat at the other end of the table, eating with one hand tucked companionably under the sleeve of Renae's blouse. She wore denim bell-bottoms, a style the big girls liked, and black clogs bought with Jaclyn's allowance money. I was so proud of Jaclyn for doing that, I bragged about it.

When dinner was finished, the kids listened to their nightly warning. No clean plates, no dessert. Unfortunately, those round green things in the vegetables were slices of okra, and Adelle balked after one slippery bite. As I got up to get dessert, I saw Renae glance around, then empty the rest of Adelle's dinner onto Renae's own plate. "Adelle's done," she yelled. "She's ready for dessert."

"Kellie-Bells, did you finish your dinner?" I asked. She nodded and held her hand out for dessert.

"Where did the name Kellie-Bells come from?" Jaclyn asked.

I thought for a minute and shrugged. "I can't remember. They've been given many nicknames over the years."

"So have we—the ones the kids give us," Jaclyn said. "I'm Jaclyn, but you know they all call me Ackie. Then Renae is Nae."

Penny recited in the same singsong voice. "I'm Ube, I don't know why. Rosie is Osie."

"Marianne is Wattawa and Camille is Nommy," Jaclyn added.

They finished in unison, giggling. "And Evelyn is M and M."

"See?" Penny pulled her beeper off her belt and held it up to show everyone the last message. The beeper's digital display read O-S-I-E. That was Rosie's message for Penny.

Henry and Karley, his particular favorite, shared a bowl of ice cream, their heads close together, leaning over the dish. He spooned one spoon of ice cream for her, one for himself. The air around them was quiet. One spoon for him. One for her.

Jo-Layne, of course, had finished hers and was licking the bowl as I helped clear the table. She had a stripe of ice cream around her mouth two inches wide. Jaclyn laughed and pointed. "Mom, come see what your pigetta has done."

When Jo-Layne, who didn't realize she was about to be inspected, held her hand out for a cranberry muffin, I cried, "Excuse me! First, clean yourself up. Look at your hands! And look at that mess on the table!" Obligingly, Jo-Layne patted her hands on her cheeks and smeared the ice cream all over her face.

Jaclyn rolled her eyes and turned away. "They never get full, do they, Mom?" As Jaclyn glanced across the table at Adelle, she frowned. "What's wrong with her?"

Adelle was chewing a piece of muffin and making a terrible face. There were tears in her eyes.

Jaclyn reached over and poked through the rest of the muffin. "What's in this? Cranberries?" She stuck her tongue out. "They're sour!"

Undaunted, Adelle reached for more muffin. "No more, you don't like it," Jaclyn cried. "Why are you eating it when you don't like it?"

While everyone was busy cleaning up dishes, Champ crumbled his muffin onto the table and swept the crumbs on the floor. He gazed around the room nonchalantly, picked up another piece of muffin, and did the same thing again.

Jaclyn spotted him and called out to me. "Mommy!"

"Would you like to mop the floor after dinner, Champ?" I asked.

Champ shook his head hard. He had no idea how lucky he was that night, though. It was time for bed, and I knew he was going to get off scot-free in all the commotion.

Dinner was over. The kitchen brigade finished dishes and trooped out of the room. Their day was winding down. Oh, they would work their regular shift tonight if they were on duty, but the busiest part of the day was over for them. Penny and I stayed behind to put the food away and wipe everything down.

The intercom buzzed. "Camille, telephone! It's that woman from Ohio again."

"I'll take it in my office."

We receive thousands of phone calls at the foundation each month, many of them exactly like the one I was about to answer. These calls are tough to deal with, every one of them demanding or devastating, or both. It's no wonder

. . . .

some of my staff burn out. The woman on the other end of the phone, the mother of a Down syndrome six-year-old, had called before and spoken with the staff, but I knew she would feel better if she talked to me. I sat down at the desk in my office and switched on the desk lamp at my elbow.

"Hi, Lee, how are you? I know you've been calling, but it's been real busy. What's happening?" I glanced around the room as I listened. The top shelf of the bookcase looked dusty.

"Who did you call there in your state? That's all you have there, just this mental health department? What about the Association for Retarded Citizens, the Arc? Well, you need to call them." I stood up to get a closer look at the bookshelf. Yes, that was dust up there.

"When you're unable to do anything with your life, and you're not able to work because your child requires twenty-four-hour care, that's when you call a state agency for help, but you need to be very forceful. You can't just say, 'Okay, thank you,' and hang up. You need to be persistent. And when they tell you they're backlogged, that's just to put you off. They hope you'll find other options."

I leafed through a pile of messages on my desk as the other woman talked. A crystal hanging from the desk lamp caught the light. "A waiting list!" I cried. "How could even I say we had a one-year or a five-year waiting list? No home, no institution, knows how long a waiting list is, because we never know what child is not going to survive, or what child is going to move on. What they have to do is provide more homes, more care for that child. That's when you have to go to a more political level."

While I was talking, Karley, Tiffany, and Mariah trooped into the room, like trouble looking for a place to happen. They should have been in bed. As they clamored up on the sofa, a volunteer hurried in. "You three, out, out!" she ordered in a whisper. "Mommy's busy. Come on. Tiffany, put that doll down." Tiffany smiled and ignored her, but Karley and Mariah quickly climbed down.

When Tiffany didn't move, the volunteer warned her again. "What did I say?" At her side, Karley watched. Then Karley put one hand on her hip. Even with Down syndrome, there was no mistaking her intent. Not three feet high, back rigid, face stern, she stood there and pointed one finger dramatically toward the door. "Hear me? Down!" A perfect imitation of me. I nodded thank-you to the volunteer as they trailed out of the office.

"There's a very sad way for you to do it. That's to tell them you cannot handle your daughter, and you relinquish rights. Let me tell you, you'll see how fast they come up with a home for her. Believe me, I know what you're going through. There are fifty-three thousand children in the state of Florida with nowhere to go. They're phasing out institutions that we may think are terrible, but at least they provide care."

I paused and listened for a moment. "No, you cannot be charged with neglect if you say with a sane mind, 'I cannot take care of my child, and I will relinquish my rights.' They cannot . . ."

"Money?" I asked with a laugh. "What money? See, that's another whole issue with your daughter. Here in Florida the ones whose adoptions aren't finalized get Social Security and Medicaid. Wait, not so fast, I can't just take her. You would have to come down here for an evaluation."

It was long after five o'clock on a late summer evening. I smelled fresh-cut grass as I sipped on a diet soda and listened. At some point, Sahara, my hairbrush of a dog, so small she was easy to miss, settled in my lap and fell fast asleep. I petted her as I talked. "Right, that's right. Certainly we can claim hardship for you if there's nothing else in your state. But you need to exhaust everything in Ohio. Once you've done that, then I can help you."

I heard the sound of Champ's Ninja Turtle video float in from the playroom. "Call the Arc. Call the mental health department. You can't stop there either. Call your governor's office. Let him know what's going on with this child of yours that's so totally dependent on you that you can't get out of the house."

The dog hopped off my lap as I spoke. "There's nothing I can do for you if you're not also willing to fight one hundred percent. I know it's frustrating, but you can't get frustrated. When your fight is exhausted, then I'll step in, but I'm fighting for hundreds of people every day, with the same exact issues. Please understand, I want to help you, but first, you need to help yourself!" I scooped the dog up and plopped her back on my lap.

Bill walked in, heard my tone of voice, and made a sharp U-turn out of the room.

"I understand. Is your daughter aggressive? Yes, that's when it starts. She feels the anxiety you're experiencing. One thing about Down syndrome, they have that extra sense, so she feels your anger, your tension. You know, since her birth, you've changed too. Listen, nobody ever said Down syndrome was easy. It's very difficult. While some remain docile their whole life, it may get worse as she gets older. There's a very broad spectrum of Down syndrome.

"Get her on a waiting list now. So what if they tell you it's a two-year waiting list? Say, 'Put her name down.' Call me, let me know what develops. I am sorry for what you're going through, but unfortunately that's what happens. You have had your test in life. All right, get back to me. Let me know. Keep up your fight, and I'll be behind you doing everything I can."

17 *The July Birthday Party*

❧

*E*very year I hold one of my long-standing traditions, a July birthday party for the six children born that month. This year, at a little table in the center of the playroom sat Tiffany and three others, surrounded by fidgety children in high chairs, the staff, and every volunteer. Even my sister Jo-Ann was there.

"Lights!" I cried.

As the lights dimmed, Jaclyn walked in, carrying a huge Disney World cake, covered with tiny balloons and little figures of Mickey and Minnie Mouse and ablaze with candles. The children at the table reached for the cake.

"Don't touch!" I called out.

Tiffany, Mariah, and the others at the table clasped their hands in front of them as everyone in the room sang, "Happy birthday to you . . ." Jaclyn set the cake in the center of the table, and only the children's faces, soft and shining in the candlelight, stood out in the darkened room. Tiffany and Champ, unable to contain themselves, bounced like jumping beans in their seats. The instant the song ended, they blew out every candle on the cake.

"Lights," I cried again as I elbowed my way over to Penny. "How did Champ get in there? His birthday was last May."

"Nerve," she replied dryly. "Sheer nerve."

I chuckled.

Jaclyn picked the cake up to wild applause and went around the room to the rest of the birthday children seated in their high chairs.

"Jo-Layne first."

"Happy birthday to you . . ." they chorused to Jo-Layne. When they were through and had moved on to the next child, Jo-Layne picked up a crumb that had fallen onto her tray and stuck it in her mouth. She frowned. What was all the fuss about? The crumb was so tiny it had no taste at all.

Then to Brooke. As Jaclyn lowered the cake in front of the unsuspecting birthday girl, the group sang, "Happy birthday to you . . ." They sang every line while Brooke sat in Eunice's lap and watched entranced, not believing that the cake was for her. She looked up from one face to the other, then down at the cake, mouth open, hands far apart, too surprised to clap.

Then it was Adelle's turn. Jaclyn set the cake on Adelle's high-chair tray.

"Happy birthday to you . . ." Not one word was left out. Jaclyn stuck Adelle's finger in the icing and steered it into the child's mouth. Adelle's face lit up, and she plopped her whole hand in the cake. When the laughter died down and

. . . .

her hand was licked clean, Adelle flipped her hand from front to back, checking for more.

"Marci!! Happy birthday to you . . ." As they sang, Marci, one of our handicapped adults, sat with her hands folded in her lap, grinning. She swallowed and composed herself. But she couldn't contain her grin, and it spread across her face from ear to ear.

Mariah plopped on the floor in everybody's way. "Mariah, sit down!" A wide smear of icing ran from her mouth to her ear. Where did she find icing? The cake had been hidden away, and they hadn't even cut it yet.

"Jo-Ann, stand up here next to me," I said. She and I blocked the children's view into the next room where their present, a play kitchen, waited.

"Surprise!" The children jumped up and down and hollered when they saw their gift.

The staff had wrapped every item in the little kitchen, play food, dishes, and kitchen utensils, so there would be plenty of gifts to open. As Champ reached for a gift, one of the volunteers stopped him. "No, let them open their gifts. It's not your birthday."

"No, they *all* open the gifts," I said. "All my children open gifts at every birthday." I wasn't going to have some of the children open presents while the rest of them watched. That isn't fair. Not all of them understood what was going on. Besides, even if they had understood, I still don't think it's fair. It's hard to watch somebody get a present and not get one yourself.

Tiffany lifted a big package and staggered across the room with it. "Brooke, Brooke, for you!" Tiffany was a little excited that day, and she handed the gift to Sandy. No wonder. There were people everywhere, and with all the cries and yells, wrapping paper flying everywhere, it was impossible to tell whose birthday it was.

Christopher, safe in his blue beanbag chair, waved a plastic piece of pie Jaclyn had opened for him and watched the others. Jo-Layne kept her eye glued on Champ as he unwrapped a fake hot dog. Her glance darted from his hot dog to the plastic piece of cake in her hand. Unable to resist, she bit into the fake cake, made a face, and threw it on the floor.

In the corner, Leanne smiled and quietly rocked one of the babies as she glanced around the room, not especially interested in what was going on. She was content doing exactly what she was doing.

"Okay, here's one for Woody," I cried. I laid my hand on Woody's forehead while he stared blankly at me. "My Woody Woodpecker!" I patted his cheek. "Champ, you want to help your brother?" I knew the package contained something about Champ's cherished Ninja Turtles.

Champ squatted on the floor in front of Woody to unwrap the large gift. He tore off a corner and realized instantly what it was. "Ninja!" A blanket covered with Ninja Turtles! He squatted again, tore off a small piece of paper, stood up, and ran over to hand the piece of paper to Renae. He did this over and over, opening the gift in inches. In a wide-striped yellow-and-black shirt, tearing back and forth from Renae to the gift, he looked like a frantic bumblebee.

"Woody!" Jaclyn yelled. "We forgot to sing 'Happy Birthday' to Woody."

Woody was born profoundly handicapped, without hope for recovery. Like Mariah, he was doomed to live out his days as a hospital boarder patient. But Woody's parents refused to accept that, and they called me.

When we met, his mother had that stunned, dazed look anguished parents wear. She cried as she explained how they felt about him. All they wanted was a life for their son. If they chose not to provide it, in spite of their families' objections, they were prepared to live with that decision. But they refused to let him stay in that hospital. Would I take him?

When I first met Woody, I saw a baby with thick blond hair, lying in a hospital crib, tube-fed, and unaware of his surroundings. How could I not want him? If there was any chance that he would survive with us, why should he live out his life pathetically in a hospital? That went against everything I believe in.

So, after the necessary paperwork was done, and I had the parents' authorization, I simply removed Woody's feeding tube and took him home. I didn't play God and decide his future. I taught him how to suck and take a bottle. When that tube came out, Woody could have fulfilled his doctor's prognosis and died. But he didn't.

Later, when his mother told me that I had saved his life, I was quick to answer.

"No, that isn't so. Woody chose to live. All I did was support his decision."

"*H*appy birthday to you . . ." everyone sang to Woody. He was five years old.

Jaclyn grabbed the cake right out from under the hands of the volunteers who were cutting it and hurried over to him.

"Happy birthday to you . . ." the room chorused as Jaclyn swiped at the cake with her little finger and stuck the icing in Woody's mouth.

Severely handicapped, oblivious to the celebration of his birthday, oblivious to the party, the music, the people here —oblivious to me and to his mother who had birthed him and loved him—Woody sucked at the icing's sweet taste and opened his mouth for more.

After the party, I made my usual rounds, checking the children. Searching for the sniffles or a fever, listening for a croupy cough or a breathing problem.

"Hi, Christopher. You're a big boy, aren't you?" He was lying in the center of the room in an overstuffed beanbag chair. When I spoke to him, his eyes searched the room, and he began to cry. But he didn't move his head. From the eyebrows down, he is a beautiful, finely drawn three-year old. From the forehead up, he is grossly, hugely malformed. His head weighs fifteen pounds.

"Christopher! Look! Mommy's here." I leaned over him

and repeated myself until I got his attention. Once his eyes fixed on my face, his gaze never wavered.

He grimaced and pulled at his shirt. "What's wrong?" I asked. Something was hurting him. "I'll be right back. I'll go find Daddy."

When Christopher's mother was four months pregnant, she and her husband learned through an ultrasound test that they were going to have twins. They also learned that there was a problem. For five months, they waited, and when the children were born, Christopher's twin sister was normal and healthy. Christopher, however, was born hydrocephalic. Better known as water on the brain, it is a condition characterized by too much fluid in the skull, resulting in deterioration of the brain.

His parents and I met at my office to discuss what to do. What was the best thing for him? The doctors held little hope for his survival. They didn't even think he would roll over or sit up. His parents wanted a safe place for him to live for as long as he was alive. A "no code" order had already been issued at the hospital. Christopher was not to be resuscitated if he stopped breathing. We agreed I would bring him home to live, and they would visit often.

It was an awful ordeal for them. Not only did they have the trauma of Christopher's birth, but they also had a new baby to care for and two other children at home who still didn't understand. Their five-year-old asked repeatedly why Christopher wasn't coming home.

When I picked him up at the hospital, I met with the organ donor unit. They gave me their telephone number to place in Christopher's file, so I would have it near me when I needed it. I stuck it in his folder like they suggested, but I never wanted to see it again.

Christopher came home like a little prince to a water mattress, a sheepskin, a new rubber doughnut for his head, and a down comforter. And, in what seemed like only the blink of an eye, he was three years old. We taught him exercises to strengthen his neck and shoulder muscles to support the weight of his head, and while he isn't walking yet, he is sitting up.

He's our barometer too. Rosie uses Christopher to gauge how well potential employees are going to fit in. If Christopher's appearance sends them running, this is not the job for them.

I heard Christopher wail loudly as I walked back into the room with Mike. Without a fuss, Mike lifted him to the medical station, and, within minutes, Christopher had been examined, instructions written for the rash on his chest, a staff member sent to make an appointment with a skin specialist, and Christopher deposited back in his beanbag chair. There was no alarm, no outcry, no unusual movement or sound. It is amazing how quickly and quietly everyone deals with the problems. You can't go wrong in any decision you make about these children as long as the child and the child's needs come first.

One day I was talking on the phone with a Canadian man interested in giving some land to the foundation. Everyone knew it was an important call, but in the middle of my conversation, Bill rushed into the office and thrust a phone message under my nose.

"The school called. Christopher has a suspicious mark on his leg, and they're going to report you to Health and Rehabilitative Services. But, before they do, they want someone to go down there and see Christopher's leg."

Christopher is very strong, so strong that I don't allow our female employees to pick him up, because he pinches them hard enough to leave black-and-blue marks. That morning, as the staff walked the kids to the bus stop, Henry had carried Christopher in his arms. Suddenly, Christopher reached for the gold chain around Henry's neck. When Henry tried to stop him from pulling it off, Christopher jerked back so quickly that the weight of his head started to pull him out of Henry's arms. Naturally, Henry held on tight to the boy's legs to keep him from falling, and left a mark on one leg.

I took Henry aside before I went to the school. "You have to come with me. If they file a report on you, you will never be allowed to work in this field again. You will never be allowed into medical school. This is very important to you, Henry. You must come with me."

He nervously agreed.

Usually when I visit the school, the reception is warm and friendly. Not that day. Henry and I were completely ignored.

Totally rebuffed. When I met with a school official, I asked immediately what was going on.

"Christopher has a mark, a bruise, on his leg," the official said, "but, because I know it's you, I waited to report it."

I stared at the man, my face stone. "First of all, you are wrong. Not in what you think about me, but in what you did. If you suspected, even for a moment, that the mark on my child's leg was something you thought I did, or something my staff did, you were supposed to go right to HRS, and you know it. You are not supposed to call me and wait until I get here."

For ten minutes, I listened as he stammered and tried to explain. Then I brushed his words aside. There was nothing he could say to defend what he had done. He knew he had been wrong.

I stood up. "I want to see the teacher who reported this to you."

The meeting with her was just as brief.

"You know me! I have a lot of children in this school. You know I don't beat them. If I did, you would have found marks on them long ago. And you know it. You and I are both childcare professionals, and you know I have never abused one of my children."

All children—adopted kids, children in the foster-parent system, and children living at home with their own parents—need to be protected by all of us. Physicians, police, as well as schools and public agencies, have the eyes to spot abuse

. . . .

and the power to do something about it. I wouldn't want it any other way.

The school staff was lucky I didn't report them then or on another occasion. I still shudder when I think of the day they took Christopher outside for playtime and laid him on the ground instead of leaving him in his wheelchair. They knew he couldn't get up by himself. Yet they didn't look where they put him, and Christopher spent his playtime lying on a mound of red fire ants. We counted the bites. He was bitten twenty-seven times.

That afternoon, back at the foundation, I watched Christopher as he cried, an angry, pay-attention-to-me cry. Henry moved him out of the beanbag chair into the center of the room, and it quieted him. Christopher preferred the floor. He had grown adept at rotating his body and opening cabinet doors and drawers with his feet while his head remained still. Furniture got dinged and scratched, but I couldn't complain. Christopher was one of our miracles. Each time he did something, it was a triumph for every one of us. Doctors still say to this day that his life expectancy is very poor. They're the same doctors who said he would never sit up. But look at him now. By this time next year, he'll be walking. I'm sure of it.

18 The Press

❧

*I*t was the day before Thanksgiving, and the house teemed with reporters, children, staff members, and the special needs adults. Television cameramen, still photographers, and assistants with portable phones swarmed all over the place. It happens several times every year. We are one of those holiday human interest events that people love to hear about.

As they waited to interview me, the press watched our daily reunion. The little kids, alone with the staff all day while the big kids went to school, waited eagerly every afternoon for their brothers and sisters to come home. Even Christopher, self-involved and demanding, fretted more than usual when the other kids weren't around. This day was not any different from any other one. As soon as the homebound toddlers heard the school bus, they practically knocked each other down, racing for the door.

The reporters laughed as the kids dashed to each other, jubilant at being together. Delight lit their faces as they yelled and crooned hellos, patted each other on the back and swapped rough wet kisses. Bumping noses, bumping foreheads, stumbling and stepping on each other's feet, they hugged clumsy hugs. Their faces shone.

When they spotted me, the excitement rose. Not content with hugs, they tumbled all over me, jumping up excitedly and clambering over one another to get to me. They shoved and scuffled and flew one by one into my arms. It happened all the time. Every time I entered a room, they held their arms up to me. Talk about rewards! What more did I need?

With as much sweet tenderness in her voice as Wendy, my question woman, could muster, she bent over to kiss Brooke on the cheek. "I miss you, I miss you." This grown woman was almost shy at the reunion. Nearby, Kyle piled into Patty's lap for hugs and safety as he watched the rest of the children. He was wearing his black sandals decorated with red baseball mitts for the occasion. Mariah was congested today, and she coughed constantly. The staff chased her with tissues but couldn't keep up with her nose as it ran all over her face. Seth and Rick, oblivious to the crowd, strummed a toy guitar on the couch as a television camera recorded the event. They didn't notice.

Tiffany and two other girls ignored the reporters, grabbed favorite puzzles, and plunked down in the middle of all the commotion. Champ joined four brothers and sisters at the plastic picnic table in the dining room for a game, munchkins at dinner. When Renae walked in, Tiffany yelled and rushed to her. Unable to hide her pleasure, my sophisticated teenager opened her arms and scooped Tiffany up for a long hug. Poise and strangers with cameras were forgotten as Renae buried her face in Tiffany's neck.

Mariah rushed over to a reporter who was seated away from the hubbub, trying to take some notes. She jabbed at the woman's notepad with her finger. Not satisfied, she tried to pull the pad out of the woman's hands.

"Oh, no, you can't have that. No, wait a minute. I said . . ."

Finally, Mariah snatched the pad out of her hands. The reporter grabbed it back. In seconds, they were in a tug of war.

"So what do you think of all this?" I asked Brooke as I lifted her to the changing table.

Brooke stuck her tongue out at me.

I shook my finger under her nose. "Brooke Geraldi! What have I told you about sticking your tongue out at people?"

Brooke, a wise child, popped her tongue back in her mouth.

Across the room, I heard a photographer ask a visitor, "Are you anyone?" He stammered when he heard himself. "I, I mean, are you with the group?" When she shook her head, he moved away quickly.

A skinny woman hurried in late and wondered out loud, "Is this all of the Geraldis?"

"Are there more?" the man next to her asked in a loud voice, shocked.

"This is it," I called to him, laughing at the expression on his face.

A close-shaven representative from our mortgage company squatted in a corner and watched as child after child raced by him. "Pssst!" he called, chuckling to himself at the chaos. He crooked his finger and beckoned to one of the children. "Pssst." He wasn't any different than anyone else here. He just wanted someone to play with.

The noise level rose.

A young woman with an expensive cerise blouse sought Champ out. Because he was both outrageous and outgoing, Champ was popular with reporters. As she squatted down on her haunches and shuffled toward him, she gestured for her cameraman to follow. He hunkered down and shuffled after her, both unaware of how they looked.

One reporter sitting in a chair taking notes glanced up to see Brooke walk away with one of the reporter's shoes on her foot. On the floor beside the woman's chair was one of Brooke's shoes in exchange.

Before the press got there, I didn't stop to freshen my makeup or comb my hair. There wasn't enough time. That wasn't too important for me anyway.

When I saw Kyle snatch a toy out of Mariah's hand, I went over to him. "Excuse me, Kyle Geraldi, what are you doing?" Kyle looked up at me with the face of an angel and gave the toy back to his sister.

"How do you like this great big family?" a reporter asked Leanne. The commotion and excitement made Leanne's answer more difficult to understand than usual. The man's forehead knotted in confusion, and he only pretended to write on his piece of paper.

Another reporter asked Rick what Champ's name was.

"Champ," Rick answered shortly.

The reporter frowned. "Champ?"

"Champ!" Rick replied again.

The reporter turned to the first person he saw. It was Tricia, one of the special needs adults. "Is he serious?"

"Dead serious," she replied tonelessly, her face expressionless. She sounded like Dracula.

He glanced from Rick to Tricia, certain they were putting him on, and waited for one of them to laugh. When they didn't, he smiled foolishly and hustled away.

Dozens of pictures, hundreds of feet of film later, the temperature and humidity in the room had risen. But most of the TV people stood around slim and cool, aware of their hair and their posture. There were now thirty-one people in the room and more in the foyer. When Adelle and a reporter asked me a question at the same time, I was tired enough to answer my daughter's question first. It was two thirty in the afternoon, and the staff and I had been up since sunrise. We glanced at one another as we waited for the press to finish. Even the children were starting to get cranky.

In the center of the room, Courtney and Tiffany tussled over an empty baby carriage while Patty and I watched.

"Tiffany's still having a hard time?" I asked.

"She's really a handful, eh?" Patty said.

Tiffany marched out of the room.

"Tiffany!" I cried. When the child refused to stop, I called her again and pointed to the floor beside me. "Come and sit here, please."

She ignored me.

"Excuse me?" I said softly. My words were a signal. Tiffany turned and moved grudgingly toward me. "Yes, that's right." My voice was firm as I pointed again to the floor. "Come and sit here. Thank you."

"Now look at Courtney," I said. Courtney sat on the floor with her back to me, ignoring me. "Mommy's here, Courtney. Come sit with me."

Courtney didn't budge, her little back rigid.

"She's mad because I wasn't here all day yesterday. Courtney, come give Mommy a kiss." Minutes later, with a lot of coaxing, Courtney relented and let me hug her.

A camera crew coaxed me to sit on the floor, and soon I was surrounded by the children. Champ danced up and down, grabbed me for a hug, then turned around and searched the room as if he had some "hug" left over and was looking for someone to give it to.

The head reporter crouched down on the floor with me, held a microphone in front of me, and asked his questions. "They always act like that whenever they see you? You must be—" Before he finished his question, Karley grabbed the microphone and stuck it in her mouth.

While we wrestled that away from her, Champ walked in front of the camera. "Easy, fella," the cameraman called. Champ, intent on getting wherever he was going, ignored him, and the man shrugged, laughed easily, and videotaped around him. He must have been a father.

A local newscaster, tan and lean in his custom-fitted shirt, was striding back and forth confidently, clearly accustomed to moving among people he didn't know, but oblivious to the clean diaper he was carrying in his hand.

The formal interviewing began.

19 *Christmas*

❦

*E*ven though holidays mean more work, they're my favorite time of year. No, that isn't quite right. Getting a new child is my favorite time, but holidays run a close second. And tonight was exciting! Some of the children were starring in the school Christmas play. Brooke, Courtney, Karley, and Kellie-Ann sat side by side, lined up together on the hearth in matching red sweaters and red pants with red-and-green plaid bows in their hair. They were going to be Santa's elves in tonight's play.

"Where are we going tonight, Jaclyn?" Rosie asked, knowing all the children's eyes were on her.

"I don't know where we're going." Jaclyn lifted Karley onto her lap. "Karley, do you know where?"

Karley thought about it a moment before she answered. "Indachurch."

Jaclyn nodded wisely and turned to Rosie. "She said we are going to a play."

"And who's in the play?"

. . . .

"ME, ME," all of them yelled, waving their arms wildly and wriggling in their seats.

"Let's practice," Rosie said. She pointed to Brooke. "And the first elf said?"

Brooke held her hand to her forehead and mumbled quietly.

Rosie couldn't understand, so she repeated the prompt. "And the first elf said?"

Brooke smiled her baggy-eyed smile and swallowed her line again.

"What?" Jaclyn asked. "Brookie, you know I don't understand a word of that, don't you?"

Brooke just nodded and smiled.

Rosie rolled her eyes at Jaclyn and turned to Karley. "All right, Karley, you're next. Here we go. And the second elf said?"

Karley made a fist, stuck her finger in the middle of it, and whispered her line so softly you couldn't hear one syllable.

"What?" Jaclyn cried.

"Hey, you two," I called from across the room. "So much for rehearsal."

That night the kids waited onstage for the play to begin. The curtain was still open, so the audience watched the pre-play activities with amusement. The children playing elves wore Santa Claus stocking caps, green pointed collars decorated with bells, and dark green pointy-toed elf shoes. Still spiffy and neat, no one wrinkled or dirty yet, they were adorable. Only Karley had a problem. Her hat was too big, and

. . . .

it had slipped so far over one eye that she had to look up to see, but she didn't mind. She was happy as a clam. On the floor in front of her, Brooke just noticed that she had a bell on the end of her shoe. She fingered it, puzzled. That seemed a very strange place for a bell.

In the audience, I laughed out loud as I watched them. Henry, Mike, and Jaclyn sat with me. Nervous for the children, I was glad they were there. The curtain closed for a moment, then parted to applause. The Christmas performance began.

A little boy stood center stage, reading the opening lines of the first skit. "Five little elves sitting in the sleigh . . ."

Behind him, Karley and Brooke stood in a cardboard sleigh with three other elves. Karley's hat now hung below her nose. I sighed. I knew she couldn't see a thing. Each child mumbled their lines, no one understood a word, and before you knew it, the skit was over. As the act ended, Karley finally succeeded in pulling her hat up. She was just in time to see the back of the curtain as it closed.

During the next act, I saw Tiffany in the wings while a young girl with skinny legs, dressed as a giant silver star, stood in a spotlight and sang. She wasn't very good, but Tiffany watched mesmerized, loving every minute of it.

Jaclyn tugged at my sleeve and pointed toward the stage. "Look!" There was Mariah, all dressed up in her Christmas dress, sneaking around behind the singer. From the disagreeable look on Mariah's face, she didn't like the singer either.

In the last skit, Karley sat on the floor hatless. Her only

job for the rest of the evening was to listen. At the end of the play, everyone lined up for bows. Karley's row stepped forward holding hands and bowed from the waist like seasoned actors. Karley bent over to take her bow with the others, but when she heard the applause, she froze. The other children raised their heads and stood up straight. Karley didn't move.

Jaclyn called softly. "Pssst, Karley. Get up now. Stand up."

Karley didn't move. The boy on her right tugged at her hand. She still didn't move. Finally, a teacher in the wings beckoned to them, and the group moved offstage in a line, holding hands, pulling Karley along with them like a sack of potatoes. I watched them haul my daughter offstage. She was smiling her heart out, still in the middle of her bow, bent over like she was having back spasms.

With nights like that to celebrate and remember, my spirits don't get low very often. Besides, only a few things in life upset me—dealing with the state bureaucracy, living with society's lack of compassion for my children, and the most important one of all, handling the stress when one of the children is hospitalized. But when I do get down, there are two stories that always help.

It was just after Christmas several years ago. The staff and I had been active in the community during the holidays, doing respite and daycare here at the foundation, and helping at some of the other institutions. But when it came to being on the receiving end, my staff had been completely forgotten. Only one present arrived, a can of chocolate-covered pretzels.

I was used to the Down syndrome adults being forgotten at Christmas. I buy their gifts anyway, and that's fine. They get so excited it's worth every penny just to watch them receive a present. But everybody buys gifts for the little children. We have so many Santas hanging around our house at Christmas that my children think he's a close friend.

"Oh, hi, Santa," they say, like it's no big deal.

When we didn't receive anything that year, I didn't care for myself, but the staff deserved more than a can of pretzels. Half the time, I was upset. The other half of the time, I was depressed. We work with hundreds of families. We never charge. Do they think I owe it to them? I spend Mike's money, and what do we get in return? I don't ask for thank-yous, but everyone likes to feel appreciated. Besides, the foundation was running us into the ground financially.

Was it me? Was it something I was doing wrong? I finally told Jo-Ann we were going to change. I was going to start doing things differently. "I don't know what, and I don't know how, but I'll know when my sign comes." Inside though, I was doubting myself.

A few days later, Mike and I were asked to speak on a new call-in radio show on WMCU. The topic for the show was abortion. The radio station pointed out that it was a new show on a small station, and they hoped we would understand that there might not be many calls. That was fine.

. . . .

As Mike and I sat in the broadcasting booth the night of the show, a technician went over the procedures with us and explained the various rules. We were instructed when to speak and when not to. We were shown how to unclip and quickly remove our mikes if we needed to cough or sneeze.

"Good evening, and welcome to the Tuesday evening MCC forum entitled *Perspective.*"

The two hosts asked the usual questions. How did we meet? What were the latest statistics on Down syndrome? Initially, the responses were Mike's. When I was asked a direct question, I answered, but I knew I sounded depressed. I tried to act enthusiastic, but it was impossible. When the host asked about our summer camp, I heard myself complaining.

"We took twenty children to camp last summer and said donations only. Only one family donated. Some came with nothing for their child, and it ended up costing us thousands of dollars. AIDS babies get funding, crack babies get funding, but Down syndrome children get no funding. Our children don't get Medicaid or Social Security. So many support groups don't last either. How come they just fall by the wayside? I don't understand."

When one of the hosts asked what I looked for in volunteers, I replied automatically, "Dedicated people who will love the children and enjoy being with them. That's all."

After a few minutes of discussion, the station opened the phone lines for audience calls. I checked my watch and rolled my eyes at Mike. I was sure the time was going to drag.

"Remember audience, tonight's topic is abortion." The

first line lit up. The host nodded at us, pleased to get at least one phone call. "Good evening, you're on the air."

"Hi, my name is Michael, and I want to brag on these two people. My wife and I had a Down child four years ago. The Geraldis might remember us. They're the ones who lifted us up and brought us through that traumatic experience. This child has been the blessing of our lives, and whatever the Geraldis need, or whatever they want, they deserve to have."

"We remember you, Michael," I said. My voice quivered, and I tried to take the darned microphone off, so the audience wouldn't hear me. I was so touched at his call that I was afraid I was going to cry. "Thank you."

Seconds later, the next line lit up. "Hi, my name is Gwen. I can say wonderful things about them too. They take care of my son."

Oh my God, it was Gwen. I couldn't believe it. Mike was grinning all over the place, and I was still trying to get the mike off. How did you unhook the thing? I must have made some sort of noise on the air, because Gwen noticed. "Is that them laughing?"

"We're not laughing, Gwen," I replied. By now, it was obvious that I was crying. Believe me, I never let people see me cry.

"Wait a minute," Gwen said, as her own voice cracked. There was a long pause before she continued. "My child was in the hospital for three months. The doctors told me he was going to die. The Geraldis helped me get him out of there, and now he's seventeen months old. They worked out the money, so I got to keep him. And he's wonderful."

For the next ninety minutes, abortion, the evening's topic, was never discussed as calls poured into the station.

"Never set limits on your child, she told me," one caller said. I didn't recognize the voice.

"They gave me strength," another caller offered.

"Camille said always believe that God is the giver of good gifts."

*T*hat radio show was my sign. After that show I realized I have to do this because I want to, not because I want to get thanked. And besides, the children thank me—the children thank me all the time.

The second incident happened shortly after Jo-Layne's open-heart surgery. Just home from a year in the hospital, Jo-Layne was sleeping in my bedroom, hooked up to a heart monitor. In the rest of the house, I was entertaining hundreds of people. It had only been a few days since her surgery, and she was still very ill, but the celebration was in her honor. Our friends and family were also there to witness the christening of our newest child.

During the party, I slipped away to look in on Jo-Layne. As I leaned over her crib to check the monitor, I heard voices in the bedroom doorway behind me. Two Baptist ministers and a Catholic priest were chatting to each other while they watched me tend to Jo-Layne.

"How can you do all this?" the priest asked, gesturing first to the sick baby and then out to the party.

"Well, Father, I'm very lucky. If the children sleep, I sleep, of course. But God blessed me with not needing a lot of sleep. Before this, when I was just a doctor's wife, I did two things. I went to luncheons and I slept," I said with a chuckle. "That's all I did. I guess I was getting ready for all these years. Now I don't need any sleep."

"No, that's not it," one of the ministers said as he watched me. "Mother Teresa never needed much sleep either."

That's my favorite story. Can you imagine, comparing me to Mother Teresa!

Karley played a big part last Christmas too. She was on the Geraldi thank-you committee for a special gift we had received. Every classroom in Pinewood Acres, an elementary school near us, drew the name of one of our children, and the school children bought a Christmas present for that name. On Christmas morning, there were so many gifts! Rosie knew ahead of time that I would be too busy to do more than write a thank-you letter, but she thought the school deserved something special.

So she took pictures of all the kids as they opened their presents. Then she made a card four feet high and glued on all their pictures. One day she took Karley and Seth, dressed in outfits they had received from the children at the school, to Pinewood Acres to give the school their thank-you card. They walked around to every class, thanked them and took their pictures. You should have seen the faces on those schoolkids.

Karley wanted to go back and thank them again. Not because etiquette was a big thing with her, but because one of the teachers had given her a cupcake.

20 *A New Baby*

🌿

When Rachael first came to the foundation in a wheelchair, she was a young, bright fourteen-year-old with cerebral palsy. Her mother had called us repeatedly for help, and each time Rosie talked to her, I explained what to say and where to send her for help. I wanted Rosie to learn how to handle these calls on her own. One day, we were working late in the office when the phone rang. Rosie was already on a call, so I answered the phone. It was Rachael's mom.

"Yes, Rosie has told me about you," I said. "What you need to do is call Developmental Services. *They* can find a group home for your daughter."

As she talked, I started to understand the situation she was in. Five minutes into the conversation, I said, "Call Developmental Services and tell them you have a home that will *possibly* consider taking her *if* you can get the funding."

Another five minutes passed. I had tears in my eyes as she explained how she couldn't handle Rachael alone anymore. She sounded desperate. "All right, I'll see her. We'll come

. . . .

and do an evaluation. Then you can call Developmental Services, and tell them you have a group home that will take her *if* they can get the funding."

At the end of the conversation, I said, "Okay, we'll take her. No, don't worry about the funding."

Rosie laughed as I hung up the phone. "Now I see why you need me and Jo-Ann and the other people in the office. No wonder they keep you away from the phones. They need to fend everybody off. If we didn't, you'd have a million children here. You cannot say no to anyone."

Rosie didn't know the half of it. In two hours, a new baby was supposed to arrive.

On the way to the West Palm Beach Airport, the one time I wanted Bill to hurry, he drove like a snail. Any other night, we'd be in the wrong lane, tearing down the road a million miles an hour. Here it was after eight, pouring buckets outside, and we were still thirty minutes from the airport.

Ahead of us, the headlights shimmered off the slick highway. Jaclyn, Bill, and I were meeting the parents of a week-old infant. The family was flying in from Texas, handing their baby girl over to us at the airport, then turning right around and flying back home that night.

"Come on, Mom, just this one time," Jaclyn pleaded, fussing with one of those little Troll figures, the kind with long purple hair. "Please, just this once, can I name the baby?" It was not the first time that night she had asked me the same question.

. . . .

"I'll name the baby," I said. "You know I always name the girls. Now, please fix your hair." I crossed my legs and nervously swung one foot back and forth.

"Yeah, but what are you going to call it?" Jaclyn asked as she edged forward on the seat. She couldn't sit still either. "I know, I know, how about Angela? No? Adelle? No! That's dumb. We already have an Adelle." She laughed at herself, embarrassed.

"Noel is nice," I mused out loud, "Noel," I said again, drawing the name out slow, testing its sound.

"You could name the baby Spot." Bill laughed nervously as he glanced at me in the rearview mirror. Aware that I was always on edge before I picked up a new child, he was trying to put me at ease. We were all anxious, nothing would have helped that night. The car hummed with tension.

"Bill, we're meeting Jo-Ann at the airport. She has all the papers the parents need to sign."

"Name her Spot?" Jaclyn cried. "My new little sister! Are you crazy? I know, how about Party Hearty!" She collapsed in giggles, far less nervous than the grown-ups, but still so excited, her voice was shrill. It was Christmas for her.

I shushed them, too distracted to listen to their chatter. I seldom use the birth name the parents give to a child. I always explain to them that the babies are given another name when they come into the Geraldi home as adopted children. It is very difficult for the parents to understand that their time of devastation and hurt is a time of joy and excitement for us. And naming these babies is one of the ways I bond with them.

When we entered the airport, the first thing I did was scan the arrival board for the flight. The plane was late. We waited for half an hour, then an hour. I stood in front of the airport window, gazing through my reflection to the tarmac below. When the flight was finally announced, no one moved except Jaclyn. She headed right for the door to the jetway, bouncing up and down on the balls of her feet. I watched and waited. One by one, the passengers hurried through the double doors that led from the jetway to the waiting room, until surely everyone had to be off the plane. Finally, a flight attendant towing his luggage behind him strolled through the door.

"Where are they? They must have missed the flight," Bill said.

"They might have," I said, surprised. "If they aren't on this flight, we'll call."

Jaclyn flitted around us. "Look! More stewardesses are leaving. This is the right plane, isn't it?"

"Shhh!" I told her. "Be still! You're making me crazy." I couldn't hear myself think.

A young couple with a baby walked slowly through the doors.

"That's them! Is that them?" Jaclyn cried and pointed toward the jetway.

"I don't think so. Don't point," I replied as I grabbed her hand. I was right. The man grinned and gestured to the baby in his wife's arms as he waved at a white-haired man standing on the other side of the room.

The doors opened again. I nudged Bill and gestured with my chin. "There."

A short, dark-haired woman carrying an infant seat walked toward us with a good-looking blond young man. In the airport's fluorescent lights, the woman's skin was yellow with fatigue. She looked as if she hadn't slept in days.

I started for the couple immediately, one hand extended, deliberately letting them think I was late. I talked nonstop to fill the awkward gaps. I had acted out this terrible moment many times.

"Hello, I'm Camille Geraldi. Are we late? I hope not. No? Good."

The man extended his hand, and I ended up greeting him first, but my attention was focused on the woman and the infant seat.

"Is this the baby?" I asked the young mother, then bent over the infant seat before anyone could answer. The baby was tiny and pink, and blond like her father. She resembled Karley when she was small. Looking up into the mother's face only inches away, I tried to draw her into conversation.

"Let's find some place to sit. The airport is really deserted tonight," I said as I put a hand lightly on her shoulder and steered her to a group of seats off to the side. "These baby clothes she has on—they're beautiful," I cried. I smiled encouragingly and sat down beside the young woman.

. . . .

The mother swallowed and smiled. "Thank you." Her eyes never changed.

Another family waiting for someone's arrival walked over and sat down in the chairs next to us.

"Come, where we can talk," I said, I picked the infant seat up from the mother's lap and ushered everyone to a more secluded corner. Jaclyn stuck to me like glue, lifting the blanket, cooing over the baby, and smiling shyly at the mother. I was glad I had brought her along. Her innocent excitement and enthusiasm eased the situation. She was a big help.

As the rest of the group settled themselves, I sat down with the infant seat on my lap.

Unsmiling, the mother reached for it, but I put my hand on her arm. "How about if I hold her for a minute? Is that all right with you?"

At the young mother's reluctant nod, I asked more questions. "Her color's good. Is she eating? She is? Good. Difficult to feed though, isn't she?"

For the first time, the mother's face took on some life. "It takes so long for her to eat."

As I explained some of the feeding quirks of Down syndrome infants, Jo-Ann walked up. She had all the documents they needed to fill out and sign before this could be official. She is also a notary, and since we needed two people to witness and sign the papers, she had brought someone with her.

"Will you be the other witness, Bill?" Jo-Ann asked. Bill hesitated for a long moment before he agreed, silently nodding his head.

She passed the papers one at a time to the parents. She worked swiftly, but there were endless pages to sign. The father barely glanced at the documents, signing everything quickly as if to get the task over with. The young mother read each page and attempted to understand every word. She didn't ask her husband or anyone else to explain anything.

The rain drummed hard on the huge window behind us. Occasionally, a security guard standing on the other side of the room glanced at us. The husband was good looking in a spoiled peacock sort of way. Blond hair, full lower lip, tight, light-colored pants, so tight you could see his underwear line. His wife wore no makeup and was dressed in a simple black dress that fit snugly over her belly. Empty of tears, her face was dazed, paralyzed as if she had been hit and not yet fallen down.

The young man leaned forward, his elbows on his knees, and told me about another adoption place they had looked at in Texas. "It was too close. My wife wanted to visit the baby every month. I said, 'What? Are you nuts?'"

The mother sitting tight to my side whispered something to me. "Of course, if you want, of course, I will call you every day," I replied. She laid her hand on the baby's cheek, afraid like so many parents had been that I would pass this baby on to someone else, so scared that she would never see her again.

I answered her unasked question, our faces only inches apart, so close I could feel her breath on my cheek. "This baby will never, ever leave me, I can promise you that. Oh, I've reversed adoptions too. We allow everything. Our foundation is very different." I stared directly into the mother's eyes with every word, trying hard to convince her, the same way I spoke to the children, creating a link between us, wishing, willing her to trust me. But it was easy to understand why she was still skeptical.

As she signed the papers, I lifted the baby and checked her face carefully. "I know you haven't gotten the genetic test results back yet, but from what I can see, it's definitely Down syndrome." I weighed my words carefully, but I never took my eyes off the infant as I gave it the bottle I had found in the infant seat. "Hear that snorting? That's a symptom. It's not a noise a baby ordinarily makes."

The man leaned toward me again and described his efforts to learn more about his daughter's condition. "Right after she was born, I went here, I went there. I was everywhere. I did this, I did that." He waved his hand and watched my face. "My family, my whole family was with me, saying you can't do this. You can't keep this baby."

I replied agreeably, "Listen, sometimes you can't do it. Believe me, I understand." I did. I meant every word. This man was grieving too, in his own way. Who was I to say he was wrong not to want this child? What I did know was this couple would have enough to deal with between them.

To the mother, I offered what comfort I could. "Her clothes are really beautiful. You should see the way I get these children sometimes. Nothing but a diaper. I always bring a new outfit with me just in case." I patted the diaper bag at my side.

There was no reaction on her face as she quietly said, "Her

name is Darlene. Will you call her Darlene?" She didn't cry, but the look in her eyes broke my heart.

"No, I'm sorry," I said gently but firmly. "We already have a Darlene."

"I see," the woman said, her eyes dull.

"You can call me anytime," I said. The mother opened her mouth to speak. I knew what she was going to ask. "Yes, I will call you every day, I promise. I will kiss her for you each morning, and when she cries at night, I will rock her."

Later as we gathered our things and said good-bye, I laid my hand on her arm. "Remember, you will never forget this baby. Remember that."

She hugged me so fiercely that it hurt. I understood. She was clinging to this one last link to her child. I hugged her back just as hard, then turned and quickly walked away.

On the drive home, the baby slept on the seat beside me in the infant bed its parents had left. I stared at the rain through the side window, one hand on the baby. "That wasn't too bad. I hate these meetings. Nothing makes them easy. You think I don't know how hard it is on the parents. I always want to get it over with. Don't you, Jaclyn?"

Jaclyn nodded and leaned over the back of the seat to talk to Bill. As they chatted, using their words to unwind, my thoughts dwelled on the parents. I know how badly that mother wanted me to call the baby Darlene, but I already have a daughter named Darlene. She didn't understand the demand she was making. I have to rename the baby. I bond more quickly with an infant when I give it a name. It's strange.

. . . .

Even though they give their children to me, parents still make demands.

No matter what time that mother got home that night, she would call me. You can tell. The truly devastated ones call within the first couple of hours. Some of them, though, literally walk away from their children. They never call again.

I stared at the baby as she slept and caught myself wondering how a parent could give up a child. That's a simple trap to fall into. It is easy for us to judge the actions of other people—and difficult to know how we would react in the same situation. I always remind myself that I have never given birth to a handicapped baby. I have never been in that unique position. I *think* I know what I would do, but how can I be sure? I can't. No one can.

There are things, however, that I'll never understand. Most parents don't even give us a dollar, let alone a bottle of formula. Yet some don't decide to relinquish their rights for two or three years. The children live with me as if I'm a glorified babysitter, and we're just a convenience. Sometimes, when I pick a new child up, it's nude. Bare assed. That's an outrage, not because I have to supply the clothing, but because a parent doesn't care enough to clothe the child.

Some days I can't get anything done. Parents who are traumatized by what has happened call or stop by the foundation to talk. Once parents are over their initial anguish, they need to learn to stand on their own. It empowers them. I can't be there forever. There are hundreds of other parents with a Down syndrome baby who need help.

I was tired, and as the glare of the headlights washed over us again and again, I felt drained.

I smiled wearily at the baby, sound asleep on her stomach, and remembered other parents. I have a special relationship with seven or eight of the families that have stayed involved with their children. There is no word in the dictionary for the emotional link between us. We are unbelievably close. Oh, I'm not a saint. When a family walks away, it's easier for me. I connect more closely with the child. But when the parents stay involved, I bond with the whole family.

I meant what I said to that mother. Our foundation is *very* different.

As the car headed south, I watched the night slip by and traced circles on the baby's back. I'm not a caretaker, I'm a mother, and what matters to me is that I matter in the life of a child.

The baby stirred and opened her eyes. "Sh-h-h, go back to sleep," I whispered. "It won't be long now. We're almost home."

Epilogue

It seems as if that baby was placed in my arms at the airport only yesterday. A lot has happened since then, that's for sure. While our family has grown larger, our faith has grown stronger, and the love we share has seen us through many difficulties. The children are growing up right before my eyes. From Darlene to Angelica, they're all doing well. I never forget though that every passing day is a milestone in their complicated lives. Of course, we have had our tragedies. Derrick, Camia, and Christopher joined Joelle as angels in heaven, but we keep them alive in our hearts. As always, the family came through the bad times more closely bonded and more compassionate of others.

Jo-Layne and Matthew have survived a dozen surgeries between them. Kellie-Ann and Adelle are happy and healthy and at home after long hospital stays. Champ is learning to read, and Karley continually dazzles us with her perfect speech. Our family has nearly doubled in size. It would take another book to tell all their stories. Donovan, our youngest, two months old, has survived four major surgeries. With all his problems, he promises to be as challenging as the others. He's another fighter, and we're confident he'll flourish. Like the others, he improves our lives without even trying.

All of the children lived through chicken pox. I'm not so sure about me. We bought Calamine lotion by the gallon for that epidemic! We traded our North Carolina cabin for a bigger compound with a pond and a creek, so we could accomodate more campers. We still have the same dedicated staff, thank heaven, and a few new people who have the same amount of compassion and loyalty as the old-timers.

The foundation continues to help special-needs children and their families. We've added hospice care to our services, and we are caring for even more medically complex children than ever before. Although these children cannot survive, I will know they had a life full of love while they were here.

After the destruction from Hurricane Andrew, we painfully and slowly rebuilt our homes in a neighborhood that had become unfamiliar to us. The response we received from all over the country was phenomenal. Today, thanks to thousands of people, our houses and our lives are back together. We even have a nursery for children under two with a guest room for the families who are too afraid to care for their children alone.

Michael and I are apart more than ever, but we continue to hold on to our dream of one day having a farm. I want to know that when Michael and I are gone, our children will continue to be productive additions to society, with good self-esteem and loving hearts. They will never be a burden to their community, not if I have anything to say about it.

Oh, I've lost 250 pounds. Aren't you proud of me? All those years of lugging that fat around! Why, I can hardly imagine I put up with it. Now Carol and I working on a book about how I did it called *Anatomy's Not Destiny: Or, Your Weight Doesn't Have to be Your Fate!* (I have to admit, sometimes I have a little trouble remembering that title, so don't be surprised if we change it.) By the way, whoever said losing weight was easy? There's nothing easy about it. But if I can do it, you can, too. I'll show you how.

So as you can see, every day is still filled with excitement, worry, and challenges. And every night I pray that the next day is even brighter and that I will be blessed once again with a day as wonderful as the one before. Don't laugh, it can happen. Today, I have forty miracles.

Stay well, always think of the children first, and never stop reaching for your dreams.

Love,
Camille

Appendix A

Family Feelings

Parents and families can go through a whole gamut of feelings as they attempt to accept and deal with the discovery that their child is handicapped. The National Information Center for Children and Youth with Disabilities publishes a pamphlet that discusses some of these feelings.

DENIAL: There's really nothing wrong. He or she only needs a better teacher, more patience. I was the same way at that age.

GUILT: It's all my fault. I shouldn't have_____.

FLIGHT: We'll see another specialist, one who can cure the problem.

ANGER: Why didn't they find this out earlier? They don't even know for sure.

FEAR: Maybe it's worse than they're letting on. What if it gets worse? What can I expect from the future?

ENVY: Those other kids are okay. They can learn easily. It's not fair. Why us?

BARGAINING: Maybe if we send him to camp he will be okay. Maybe if she has some different friends . . .

DEPRESSION: I'm not a good parent. I can't help. It's hopeless.

MOURNING: She will never be the child I hoped for.

. . . .

You may have felt any or all of these emotions, in any sequence, or all at once. What is important is to reach the point where you can say, "Yes, my child has a handicap. It is only one of many things that will make my child special. We'll work with the schools and our doctor to find out how to help our child be all that he or she can be."

Appendix B

Stimulation Techniques

Some of the ways the staff and I stimulate the children are through:

1. *MUSIC.* We use any kind and all kinds played on tape decks, radios, televisions—from Beethoven to boogie-woogie, hard rock to Handel. We attend U2 concerts and clog to Irish jigs. Lying on the grass under a tree, we watch the leaves dance to old Judy Garland albums. (Penny prefers Musical Ernie and a Jeffrey television set.)
2. *TV.* It stimulates the ear and the eye. It encourages children to imitate people's actions and to copy their speech.
3. *SPEECH.* We tell the child what we're doing as we do it, connecting the expression and the movement. Whether it's pulling on a shirt, or blowing a nose, we match the action to the words. To see how difficult speaking really is for a Down syndrome child, try holding your tongue as you speak.
4. *TOUCH.* We provide plenty of tactile stimulation: plastic, metal, terry cloth, paper, Koosh balls. One of the kid's favorites is plunging their hands into a great big pan filled with cooked cold pasta, Jell-O, or pudding, followed, of course, by a bath.
5. *TASTE.* We encourage the children to explore different tastes, so we might try the sweet taste of a banana one day and the sour taste of a pickle the next. Whatever tastes are unfamiliar to them, such as they salty taste of an anchovy, are the ones we try.

6. *SMELL.* We use a great variety of smells: vinegar, molasses, vanilla, spices, pine.
7. *SIGHT.* Around the crib we hang well-defined black-and-white pictures. Over the crib we tie soft mobiles. An unbreakable mirror in the crib shows a baby its reflection.
8. *EXERCISE.* We prescribe daily exercises that a parent learns to do and performs with the child.
9. *INTERACTION.* Some of the things we do are play with, talk to, and tease the child; make big glad faces; hug and bounce, and with hands firmly on the torso, "fly" carefully and slowly through the air; look straight in the child's face and play peekaboo; make big glad faces; teach body parts; and carry the child facing away from us, so the baby can see the world.
10. *DISCIPLINE.* In a firm way we teach manners and encourage appropriate behavior. We expect good behavior. We try to guard their fragile concentration and relieve their helpless frustration. Temper your criticism.

Appendix C

Reading List for Parents

Berger, L., et al. *I Will Sing Life: Voices from the Whole in the Wall Gang Camp.* Little, Brown, 1992.

Blume, J. *It's Not the End of the World.* Dell, 1986.

Burke, C., and J. B. McDaniel. *A Special Kind of Hero.* Doubleday, 1991.

Burns, Y., and P. Gunn, ed. *Down Syndrome: Moving through Life.* Chapman and Hall, 1993.

Cicchetti, D., and M. Beeghley. *Children with Down's Syndrome: A Developmental Perspective.* Cambridge University Press, 1990.

Cunningham, C. *Down's Syndrome: An Introduction for Parents.* Brookline Books, 1988.

. . . .

Doman, G. *What To Do about Your Brain-Injured Child.* M. Evans and Co., 1991.

Featherstone, H. *A Difference in the Family: Living with a Disabled Child.* Viking Penguin, 1981.

Feuerstein, R., et al. *Don't Accept Me As I Am.* Plenum, 1988.

Hanson, M. J. *Teaching the Infant with Down Syndrome: A Guide for Parents and Professionals.* PRO ED, 1987.

Johnson, V. M., and R. A. Werner. *A Step-by-Step Learning Guide for Retarded Infants and Children.* Syracuse University Press, 1975.

Levin, T. *Rainbow of Hope: A Guide for the Special Needs Child.* Starlight Publishing Co., 1992.

Lott, I., and E. McCoy, eds. *Down's Syndrome: Today's Health Care Issues.* Wiley Liss, 1992.

Neff, P. *Tough Love: How Parents Can Deal with Drug Abuse.* Abington, 1984.

Pueschel, S. M. *A Parent's Guide to Down Syndrome: Toward a Brighter Future.* Paul H. Brookes Publishing Co., 1990.

Pueschel, S. M., and L. Steinburg. *Down Syndrome: A Comprehensive Bibliography.* Garland STPM Press, 1980.

Smith, S. L. *No Easy Answers: The Learning-Disabled Child.* Bantam, 1981.

Stray-Gundersen, K., ed. *Babies with Down Syndrome: A New Parents' Guide.* Woodbine House, 1986.

Trainer, M. *Differences in Common: Straight Talk on Mental Retardation, Down Syndrome, and Life.* Woodbine House, 1991.

Appendix D

National Resources
Organizations

Association for Children with
Down Syndrome, Inc.
2616 Martin Avenue
Bellmore, NY 11710
(516) 221-4700

Association for Children with
Retarded Mental Development
162 Fifth Avenue
New York, NY 10010
(212) 741-0100

Clearinghouse on Child Abuse
and Neglect Information
Department of Health and
Human Services
P.O. Box 1182
Washington, DC 20013-1182
(202) 251-5157
(703) 385-7565

Down Syndrome League
2964 Miranda Avenue
Alamo, CA 94507
(510) 743-1792

ERIC Clearinghouse on
Handicapped and Gifted
Children
Department of Education
1920 Association Drive
Reston, VA 22091-1589
(703) 620-3660

Federal Information Centers
For local listing, call
(301) 722-9098

National Center for Learning
Disabilities
381 Park Avenue South
Suite 1420
New York, NY 10016
(212) 545-7110

National Down Syndrome
Society
666 Broadway
New York, NY 10012-2317
(800) 221-4602
(212) 460-9330

National Easter Seal Society
230 West Monroe Street
Suite 1800
Chicago, IL 60606-4802
(800) 221-6827

National Health Information
Center
P.O. Box 1133
Washington, DC 20013-1133
(800) 336-4797

. . . .

National Information Center
for Children and Youth with
Disabilities
P.O. Box 1492
Washington, DC 20013
(703) 893-6061

National Park Guide for the
Handicapped
National Park Service
U.S. Department of the
Interior
Washington, DC 20240

Resources for Children with
Special Needs
200 Park Avenue South
New York, NY 10003
(212) 677-4650

Hotlines

Alzheimer's Association
(800) 272-3900

Child Abuse
Child Help USA
6463 Independence Avenue
Woodland Hills, CA 91367
(800) 4-A-CHILD

Newsletters

Down Syndrome News
National Down Syndrome
Congress
1605 Chantilly Drive
Suite 250
Atlanta, GA 30324-3269
(800) 232-6372

National Down Syndrome
Society Update
NDSS
666 Broadway
Suite 810
New York, NY 10012-2317